A
of the Heart

Hemophilia Social Workers' Stories of Patients and
Mentors Who Forever Changed Their Lives

Linda Gammage, MSW, LCSW
Dana Francis, MSW, Editors

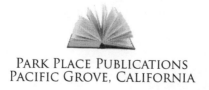

PARK PLACE PUBLICATIONS
PACIFIC GROVE, CALIFORNIA

Published by
Park Place Publications
Pacific Grove, California
www.parkplacepublications.com

Design and production by Patricia Hamilton

ISBN 13: 978-1-935530-80-0

First Edition September 2013

Printed in the United States of America

For our patients, their families, and our mentors.
We are forever grateful to you for allowing us to work with you and
share your journey.

Table of Contents

Twenty-Four Stories & A Poem

Acknowledgements

We believe a book like this is long overdue! We would like to thank all our colleagues who have contributed a story to this collection. We put out the call and many of you rose to the challenge. Some of you needed time to reflect. Some wrote about men and women who left a deep impression on you. There were tears and remembrances. Some of you wrote about children with great hope and inspiration. Others told us about important mentors. We appreciate all of you for giving of your time, digging deep into your memory and your emotions, and sharing with us the gift of a story.

We want to express our sincere appreciation to Neil Frick, Vice President for Research and Medical Information at NHF, for his generous offer to have the Stories Project book be available through HANDI. We also thank him for suggesting additional ways to distribute the book. A thank you also goes out to Morgan Johnson, Manager of Healthcare Provider Programs at NHF, for his wisdom in referring us to Neil.

We would like to thank our publisher, Patricia Hamilton, at Park Place Publications, for her expertise and her guidance as we moved through the process of creating this book. We are most grateful to her for everything she has taught us.

Linda would like to thank…

Bill: My quiet, gentle husband of 48 years; the love of my life. Your unwavering encouragement and your belief in me has been the foundation for all my endeavors. You are my unsung hero, truly "the wind beneath my wings." Thank you.

Dana: My co-editor and my "partner-in-crime." You are a deeply caring, compassionate, and remarkable social worker. You are a wonderful human being and a very valuable friend. Most importantly, we are kindred spirits. I am blessed to know you.

Social Work Colleagues: Thank you for your support and

kind words to me, not only for the Stories Project, but for any of my efforts on behalf of social workers in the bleeding disorders community. You have been, and continue to be, an inspiration to me as I remain devoted to being an advocate for our profession.

Dana would like to thank his wife, Natalie, for her editing assistance, for her enthusiastic support of creativity of all kinds, and for her endless love and patience. He would also like to thank his colleagues on the Adult Hemophilia team at UCSF Medical Center for their moral and practical support in helping this project come to fruition. Finally, and most importantly, Dana would like to thank his wonderful friend and colleague, Linda Gammage, for her incredibly focused devotion to this project. She gave tirelessly of her own time to ensure that these stories were told. Without her vision, her passion, and her boundless positive energy, this book project would never have been realized.

This project was funded by a generous grant from the Adult Hemophilia Program at the UCSF Hemophilia Treatment Center, San Francisco, CA

"The Stories Project"

"A Journey of the Heart:
Hemophilia Social Workers' Stories of Patients and
Mentors Who Forever Changed Their Lives"

The seed for this "Journey of the Heart" was planted quite inadvertently during a lunch time conversation at the Advanced Social Workers' conference in the fall of 2011. The conversation between Dana Francis and Linda Gammage began with a discussion of the length of time each had been in the bleeding disorders field.

As we talked further, thought-provoking questions arose as to why we (and many of our colleagues) have continued to work in this often challenging community. Then a second question arose – how did we survive emotionally, especially during the dark days of the HIV epidemic? Suddenly, more questions were forthcoming. Many of us work with both adult and pediatric patients. How were we able to devote the much needed time with the HIV+ patients and their families while also establishing the all-important trust relationship that would provide crucial support to the parents of the little ones? These parents were often trying to cope with their child's new diagnosis of a bleeding disorder. This diagnosis came with many questions and fears including the possibility their child could become infected with HIV.

So much was demanded of us.

As we reflected on those heart-wrenching times, we found ourselves remembering many of the patients and families who had touched and significantly impacted our lives. Those individuals, as well as our mentors, had inspired us, not only as professionals, but perhaps more importantly, as human beings.

Thus, the "Stories Project," as it was initially known, began to take shape. In talking with our social work colleagues across the country and in Canada, we realized that indeed, there were many wonderful stories that should be shared, especially with those social workers new to the bleeding disorders world. The only guideline we asked our writers to follow was to "write from the heart." We sincerely hope that as you read these enlightening, heart-warming stories, you will feel inspired and encouraged as you either begin, or continue, your own "Journey of the Heart."

Linda Gammage, MSW, LCSW
Peoria, IL
Co-Editor

Notes to the Reader

Being a social worker is an intriguing business! We toil in a profession that is chronically ill-defined. Any social worker will tell you the same thing. Our patients, and the public at large, often view us suspiciously at first. In the same way that many people think all men with hemophilia will bleed to death from a cut, many people also think all social workers simply push paper, send out welfare checks, and remove children from their homes against their parents' will. Why on earth would anyone choose such a career?

No one I know became a social worker with dreams of wealth or fame. We mostly work in obscurity and that might just be one of our best kept secrets. Often the most successful among us are the least visible. We do our best work behind the scenes. We are not "do-gooders", necessarily, but we aspire to be facilitators. We attempt to meet our patients where they reside; emotionally, economically, and socially. We assist, encourage, cajole, and provide practical and emotional support. Our goal is to help patients make changes. We are helpers but not enablers. We ask people to meet us half way. We attempt to engage them with integrity, professionalism, clear boundaries, and compassion. Then we throw in a pinch of creativity and a healthy sense of humor for good measure.

Some of the social workers who contributed to this collection of stories have been working with the bleeding disorders community for over twenty years. Others have been involved even longer. That group of social workers was baptized in the maelstrom of the AIDS epidemic. HIV and HCV, which had contaminated the patients' blood products, had a devastating impact on them and their families. AIDS changed so many things. Policy, perception, behavior...all areas of life were affected. At first, hemophilia patients felt ostracized and stigmatized because they tested positive for HIV. Homophobia and confusion were rampant. People were hiding, sick, and very afraid. Relationship dynamics between doctors and patients were forever altered. Patients began collaborating with their providers to learn as much as they could about these new viruses in an attempt to survive. It was a very fearful and chaotic time.

It was at this juncture that our patients sometimes wondered aloud if they could really trust us? Would we stick by them through this storm? What kind of people were we? What was the quality of our character? Could we handle this new intensity of their lives and their emotions? They wanted us to reveal some of our true nature so they could put their trust in us. We, in turn, realized as we faced this new frontier, we had to "lead with our humanity." Some of the more traditional "boundary issues" of our profession fell by the wayside at this time. We found ourselves summoned to people's homes and to their bedsides. Our patients and their families needed practical and emotional support. We sat and grieved with patients and family members over the enormous losses they were facing. We did our best to comfort them and to advocate for them. We were frequently asked to speak at memorial services. Everyone, patients and providers alike, were experiencing an avalanche of ongoing, unrelenting grief.

In the midst of this darkness, however, babies were being born and diagnosed with bleeding disorders as life continued on. Their parents continued to need our attention, our expertise, our emotional support, and our knowledge of community resources. We had to balance the sadness and grief we were experiencing with the hope and the energy that the children and their families required. Some of our young patients were affected by HIV. Many others were not. As social workers, we struggled to find, and maintain, the balance needed to provide service to our patients and their families. This was, and continues to be, our most important goal.

After these many years, we remember the fighters, the characters, the people who brought us joy, and those who exasperated us. There are so many people we will never forget.

Those of us who are still working in this amazing community today are apt to be in touch with a surviving wife or a parent, a sibling, or the child of a patient who has died. By keeping those memories alive and telling the stories of their lives, we continue to help patients and family members grieve and process the losses they have faced. We have learned that grieving is a lifelong journey. We have experienced the enormous challenge of sadness in our work and have tried to understand how it has both profoundly affected us, while simultaneously enhancing and strengthening our social work practice.

All of this explains why the stories in this book have been written. Some of our writers told us they could have written about many different individuals. Most of us chose just one person who touched us deeply. We hope to honor their lives with these stories. Some of us have written about adults we have known and cherished. Some of these adults have died and others are very much alive! Others wrote about a precious child with a bleeding disorder. Mentors were also honored as individuals who have shown us the grace and the power of what it means to truly be of service to others.

Most importantly, we did not want these stories to be lost. It has been our honor and our privilege to work with these individuals and their families over the years. We are proud to finally tell their stories. We know you will be moved and inspired by their individuality, their character, their tenacity, and their courage.

Dana Francis, MSW
San Francisco, California
Co-Editor

Twenty-four Stories
&
A Poem

Superman

"A hero is an ordinary individual who finds strength to persevere and endure in spite of overwhelming obstacles."
Christopher Reeve

When you hear the word "Superman," you might think of images of a cartoon superhero or maybe a movie. When I hear the word, it always makes me think of my own "Superman," a young boy with hemophilia named Jeremy.

I met Jeremy when I was a young social worker at St. Joseph's Hospital Hemophilia Treatment Center in Phoenix, Arizona in the late 1980's and early 1990's. Jeremy had severe hemophilia and, like many of the patients at that time, was also infected with HIV. During that time, HIV was a more devastating disease than it is today, and treatments were not as advanced.

When I first started working at the HTC in Phoenix in 1983, we did not have a hemophilia summer camp so we would send a few boys each year to the Colorado summer camp. In 1994, the first Arizona summer camp, Camp HONOR, was started in Prescott, Arizona by the local chapter and supported by the hemophilia treatment center.

Jeremy was a very sick boy, but he loved summer camp and would look forward to the week with much anticipation, even though he only attended for a few years. One of his favorite activities at camp was archery. We were fortunate at the time to have a local archery group, "Archers Who Care," who donated their time and equipment to make the archery sessions both fun and informative for the campers. They would come up for the entire week to run the sessions and they got to know many of our campers. Jeremy was one of their favorites. Several of the volunteers got to know him personally and kept in contact with him and his family for many years.

Another thing that Jeremy loved to do at summer camp was arts and crafts. He loved to paint and do other projects. He also liked to tell jokes and would make people laugh by dressing up in funny outfits, drawing designs on his face, or doing anything else to have fun and make both the campers and the staff laugh with, and at, him. I have a picture of us together with "Camp HONOR" painted all over his face!

In the last year of Jeremy's life, he was very ill and was almost always attached to his IV pole. I remember the last year that he went to summer camp. We were all worried that he was too sick to go, but he managed to go, even though he spent much of the time in the infirmary. Even then, he would laugh, tell jokes, and make an effort to get out and participate in activities, especially his beloved archery sessions.

In the last few months and days of Jeremy's life, one of his goals was to see the new "SpaceJam" movie that was coming out. I remember going to his house and his excitement about finally being able to see the movie, even though he was not feeling well. He made us all laugh and cry and re-evaluate what is important in life.

Before Jeremy died, one of the men from the "Archers Who Care" group made some special arrows and a quiver for Jeremy for his birthday. After Jeremy died, his father, Roger, asked the camp directors if we would set up an award in his name at camp, the "Straight Arrow Award." Every year since then, an arrow is mounted and given to the camper who exemplifies the spirit of Camp HONOR. This is voted on by all of the counselors and staff and is given to the camper who everyone feels is the most courageous and noble, in the same way Jeremy lived his life.

I still think of Jeremy shooting arrows at archery and walking around in a Superman cape, making everyone smile. He is still putting a smile on my face and reminding me of why I love camp and this community so much!

Marilyn Gradowski August, MSW, LCSW
Walnut Creek, California

M.I.A.

I had been working as a Social Worker for over ten years but was brand new to hemophilia when I met him. He was seven years old then, and although average in height and weight, there was NOTHING average about him. Born to a mother who was marginal at best, this child had seen a lot and had already been through a lot. Sagging pants, ashy skin, and hair like wool, with a bandana wrapped tight, he already looked like a baby gang member. Underneath that rough exterior, though, was a little boy who was dying to be loved.

It was my first month on the job when I was invited to Child Protective Services (CPS) for a Team Decision Making (TDM) meeting, to determine what we could do to maintain him safely in his home. Although I had spent most of my career working for CPS, (or child welfare in some capacity), it was quite strange to now be on the other side of the fence. Advocating for children is what I had spent my entire career doing, but I felt completely unprepared for this meeting and this new role.

I hadn't known this family very long and although they missed multiple medical appointments, maybe his mother had a good reason? With a long history of substance abuse and a child who had already died in her care, maybe this child should be removed? Maybe mom is clean and sober now and simply doesn't have transportation, but had anyone bothered to find out? Had anyone spoken to him or to her? How did THEY feel? What did THEY want? Well, the team decided he should remain with his mother in her home, and I decided to monitor this family a lot more closely. I decided to wrap the family in services and a lot of support.

He lived in a filthy one bedroom apartment with his mother and her abusive boyfriend in a part of town best known for drugs, gangs, and prostitution. There were beer cans and empty whisky bottles throughout the living room, alongside the garbage and clothes. The home smelled of trash, cigarettes, and marijuana. I couldn't think of one sterile place for him to receive his factor infusions. That didn't stop me from frequently visiting his home and bringing him donated food and clothes when I could. He would try to act tough, like he didn't care, but he soon called me by my name and would even ask when I would be back.

His school was seven blocks away, and when he attended, he was responsible for getting himself to and from school. *"Good afternoon, Damia. We had another school meeting to address his academics and lack of focus. He has missed 33 days of school due to his illness. Could your clinic please provide medical documentation indicating his condition and the need to miss so much school? Thank you for your help."*

I immediately went through the records. There were no reported bleeds and he was on prophylaxis. Why was he missing so much school? The only time we ever heard from his mother was when she needed food, transportation, or financial assistance. She was brought before the School Attendance Review Board (SARB) and was told that if her son did not start attending school regularly she would be fined and possibly arrested. Finally, a system that would hold her accountable as a parent... or so I thought. She simply moved him to a new school district. Problem solved for her, nothing changed for him.

She called to request a gas card so she could get him to his medical appointment. She was excited to report her father had given her $600.00 to purchase a car. Unfortunately, she could not afford the gas to put into the car. I mailed a gas card to the mom, but of course, her son never made it to his clinic appointment. I wasn't surprised. I was however shocked to learn she was being evicted from her apartment. Apparently, she hadn't paid rent. Perhaps that's how she got her new car.

Missed school, missed medical appointments, and no place to live; it was time to make the difficult decision to contact CPS. CPS knocked on the door and the family was already gone, moved to another part of the state. CPS eventually closed the case, as the family was nowhere to be found. There was no SARB hearing for this child who was not attending school. There was no police search for him, either. He was gone. No one seemed to care.

I contacted the homecare pharmacy, who had not heard from the mother. Nor had she contacted MediCal to report a change of address. She was receiving public assistance and finally reported a new address in an effort to receive her monthly cash aid. Unfortunately, they had moved too far away for me to remain involved in their case. I did alert their local HTC and let them know that he might be establishing himself as a patient. I asked them to tell him hello from me if they ever heard from the family. Months passed and I didn't hear from his mother. She never responded to my letters.

He never established himself with the new hospital and was running out of factor refills. What will become of the little boy with his whole life ahead of him, born to a mother who is marginal at best? I often thought of him. Was he doing well in school? What more could I have done to help him and his family?

And then out of nowhere the phone rang. "Hemophilia Treatment Center, Damia speaking." (pause) "Hi Damia, it's me. I was just calling to wish you a Happy Birthday!" How did he know? I was moved to tears. Just when I thought I had failed this child, he reminded me that as long as I was doing my best, I could never fail him. I was making a difference.

I will never be able to predict the future or how life's circumstances will impact an individual. All I can do is provide as much support as I can with the time that I have, and pray for the best.

Damia Dillard, MSW, LCSW
Sacramento, California

My Mentor and Teacher

I was the new social worker for the Louisiana Comprehensive Hemophilia Care Center as I stood by a young man's bed with our Nurse Coordinator, Karen Wulff. He was too young to die, yet you could tell by his emaciated state and the gray tone to his skin that he did not have much time left. Tears were streaming down Karen's face as she gently rolled him to his side and slowly rubbed his back with lotion. His body began to relax as he told her she was the best nurse anyone could have and thanked her for being there his whole life.

The sincerity of moments like this one move through me and render me in awe of this woman who has been at so many bedsides of her dying patients. She was there throughout the entire AIDS epidemic in hemophilia as it trampled this community.

How did she manage to keep on going with such dedication to these men and boys and their families? I wanted to learn from her and so began my journey with my mentor and teacher.

There have been days when I walked into the office and Karen was sitting behind her desk in scrubs because she had already been in the operating room, having arrived before dawn. Karen goes to surgery with all of our patients to administer factor and monitor their factor levels during the procedure, but that is only one reason why she does this.

How do I know? I have gone into the surgery prep room with her and have seen and felt the patient's fear as we approached his bed and then watched it melt away as Karen takes his hand to reassure him that she will be with him throughout the surgery. The trust between them is almost visible; it is the cement that binds their relationship. Karen understands the healing effect of her presence. This cannot be taught in a classroom, but it can be taught by example. Karen demonstrates this to me daily.

She explains these moments by simply sharing her ability to empathize. I don't think she realizes she does this. In addition to this empathy, she is also often accused of being overly optimistic about some of our patients who struggle with the tasks of everyday life such as simply following their medical treatment. An example would be the patient who misses his clinic appointment but calls that afternoon to tell her about the bleed he has been having for the past two days. Oh yes, she will fuss at him, but somehow he knows her words are the expression of how much she cares about him. She then advises him on what he needs to do to treat his bleed and she believes he will follow her advice.

Other team members may doubt that he will do what she recommends. When this happens, she smiles and acknowledges her gullibility, but that is not what is important. What is important is that the patient trusts her enough to call, even though he knows that he missed his appointment. He knows she will help him even if she is upset with him.

Why would this happen? Probably because there were many times when he was in pain and Karen was able to understand how bad it was and got him help quickly. He knows she is able to empathize with him and that she believes in him, even if he doesn't always do what he needs to do and especially when others don't believe in him. She is always there.

Karen is available twenty-four hours a day to the hemophilia patients in Louisiana. I don't think she has seen a movie in its entirety in the past 35 years without getting a call. The patients and their families know this and feel safe because of it. Especially new families who have just learned their child has hemophilia. Karen reassures them they can call any time and no question is unimportant.

When a child has his first bleed and the parent calls, Karen very calmly reassures them that they have time to get to the emergency room. She then calls ahead to the emergency room, explaining the situation. By doing this, the young family will hopefully be able to move through the experience more easily.

She is also a great proponent of education and knows that people have a hard time hearing what they need to know when they first get a diagnosis. So she makes sure they come back to clinic every 3 months for more education and she attends our monthly parent support group to answer any questions new parents may have.

Her availability to patients and their families is extraordinary. In fact, we joke in the office that as soon as Karen gets in, the phones ring off the hook. Karen always has large stacks of messages every time she enters the office and she will return every one that same day. She also attends all school and prison visits ensuring that staff and faculty in these facilities are well trained and know how to reach our Center. She explains that any phone call they make to our Center will be treated as though a physician is calling. This means they are high priority and everyone in our Center knows this.

She demonstrates these standards to her patients and their families, to the multi-disciplinary team, and to professionals outside of the team. Sometimes when I am on hospital visits with Karen, I am amazed at how she is able to quietly listen to a staff doctor, fellow, or resident who may have a "know-it-all" attitude that day, but truly does not understand how to treat hemophilia. She does not lose her temper or become insulted; instead she will simply explain that she has seen how a patient with the same problem in the past has gotten better when we did such and such. In a few minutes the physician is usually giving an order to a nurse on the floor to do exactly what Karen said, but he/she now looks like the one who came up with the plan.

Karen never takes credit for having given that knowledge because that is not what she is trying to accomplish. She wants her patient to receive the best treatment and she has enough skill to carefully pass the necessary information along in a way that gets her patient what he needs and saves the doctor from the embarrassment of error. Professionals from around the country call on Karen for her expertise in hemophilia treatment and she serves on numerous national nursing educational committees. She is called to give lectures both nationally and internationally, yet you would never know this by her humble approach to her daily work.

After having been a social worker for over 35 years, walking beside Karen Wulff as she visits with our patients always teaches me something new. Our patients, their families, and our staff are blessed to be in her company. She demonstrates the hallmark of mentorship.

Sue duTreil, PhD, LCSW
New Orleans, Louisiana

Gary Clark: A Friend Remembered

I became involved with hemophilia in 1971, although I didn't know it at the time. It was the beginning of a new school year and I was a freshman in high school. In just a few months, I would be 14 years old. I got to know Gary Clark that year. He was about 16, in the 11th grade, and one of the cutest boys in the whole school!

During the first week of the 1971-72 school year, we were given our class schedule. Study hall in the library for me almost first thing each morning. One morning, the door opened and there he stood. Gary. Looking around for a place to sit, he came directly to the table I shared with two of my girlfriends. We couldn't believe it! He was so cute, and he was sitting with us! He could have sat anywhere, but he sat WITH US!!!! I don't remember if we were supposed to be cool or groovy in 1971; it didn't matter, we were neither. But, our coolness factor went from negative numbers to double digits that day for sure, at least in our eyes.

Gary was tall and thin with collar length wavy brown hair. I think I have already mentioned that he was very cute but Gary was also one of the nicest guys I had ever met - and that holds true to today. He always seemed to have a smile in his eyes. Needless to say, I developed a crush on him as did most of the girls at our school.

Study hall became a lot more interesting with Gary at our table. The thing about Gary was that when he talked to us, he treated us as if we were the same age as he - not the 13 year old little dweebs we really were. He teased us, sure, but he never talked down to us. He would ask what we thought about some issue or book and I could have spent hours just talking to him, and let's be honest - looking at him. We both liked to read so the library was the perfect place for both of us. He was the first person who ever made me think about what I had read and what, if anything, I got out of it. A lifelong lesson, I would say.

I mentioned that I had a crush on Gary but it really wasn't that - I just liked him so much. He seemed magical to me. He was the kind of person who liked other people. He was a popular guy and was usually surrounded by his classmates, both girls and boys and he almost always had a girlfriend or two. Despite that, he gave some of his attention to me and because of how he talked to me and treated me, I gained a confidence in myself that I didn't even know was missing. When the school year ended, he wrote in my yearbook "to a nice girl I will always remember."

The following summer, my sister and I went to the movies with our cousin and her boyfriend. They dropped us off at the theater and then failed to pick us up. We lived about ten miles from town and didn't know what to do except to start walking home. We couldn't call our parents and rat out our cousin, but ten miles is a long walk. What else could we do? It was getting dark and as we were standing on the sidewalk, a car pulled up - it was Gary! He and a friend were out driving around when he saw me and decided to stop and say hi. He and his friend drove us home. He really was my knight in a shining Chevy (I don't know if it was really a Chevy, but it sounded good when I wrote it.)! The next year, Gary graduated from high school and that was the last I saw of him for many years, although I never forgot him.

Years passed and in 1986 I started a new job as the social worker with Kentucky's hemophilia program. I had never known anyone with hemophilia but I was so excited to be a part of this comprehensive program. I told the nurse coordinator where I grew up and she said she had a former patient with hemophilia from that county. He had moved out of the state and his name was Gary Clark. I told her I knew a Gary Clark but that he didn't have hemophilia. I did look at the chart, though, and I recognized the name of Gary's brother who was listed as a contact person. I realized I was wrong. Hemophilia had been a part of my life for a long time. I just didn't know it.

About five years passed before Gary came back into my life. He had been admitted to the hospital for bleeding but also had some complications from HIV infection. By then, HIV had taken a terrible toll on the hemophilia community and I was heartbroken that Gary and his family had to deal with it too. I called him in the hospital to see if I could visit. I was concerned that he might be uncomfortable with me being the social worker with the hemophilia center, but I need not have worried. We talked on the phone that day and I traveled to see him the next. When I walked in the room, he said, "I remember you!" We spent the afternoon with "do you remember?" and "whatever happened to?" I told him that I never knew he had hemophilia. He said, "I thought everybody knew because I was absent so much."

Gary was back at home after some years of living away. He had had different jobs, among them, a position as a nanny to a family. He never married, although he had been engaged but broke it off when he found out about the HIV infection. Now that he was beginning to show some signs of illness, he wanted to be with his family. He was very matter of fact about it. He didn't have any plans to do anything except to spend time with his family and read.

He began attending the comprehensive clinic and became friends with just about every person there. He would always bring a book to clinic so he could read while waiting to be seen but I don't think he ever got any reading done. I talked with him often and learned that what he had loved most in his adult life was working with kids. I asked him to become involved in our hemophilia summer camp, and he did! He loved camp and the kids loved him. They saw his magic right away. He treated them the same way he had treated me so long ago. He talked to them as if they were the most important people on earth. They had something to say and he wanted to hear it. Camp was a great experience for him and he was so happy to be a part of it.

On the first night of his very first camp, however, Gary was initiated by blood. He was the counselor in charge of the 6 and 7 year old boys. He had them all in bed and had settled down to read when around midnight he heard a thump. A 6 year old (with severe factor VIII deficiency) from our hemophilia center, also at camp for the first time, had fallen out of the top bunk, hitting his head a couple of times on the way down. Gary scooped him up, held a towel on the cut, and ran with him to the infirmary. The little fellow was infused and stitched up. The ambulance was coming to take him for a scan to make sure the cut was just that and nothing more. He was calm, but Gary was not. He told the little boy, "I'd go with you to the hospital little buddy, but I have to take care of these other boys to keep them from falling out of their beds." From that night on, Gary put the boys to bed and then used all the duct tape, packing tape, ACE bandages, and whatever else he could find to put around the beds so the boys didn't roll out in the middle of the night! A couple of days later, the little guy showed back up at camp, bringing Gary some peanut M&M's. He said, "I wanted to come back to camp to see Gary!"

Gary died in 1995. I saw him for the last time shortly before that. He was living with his brother in the little county where we grew up. I visited him there and spent some time just talking to him. Although I had said it before, I told him again how much he had meant to me when I was a kid and how much I appreciated what he had done for the kids with hemophilia. He said he had loved every minute of it and was glad he was able to do something to help somebody. As I left that day, I said, "save me a seat in study hall." He said, "I will."

When I was asked to contribute a story about someone who had impacted my life, I thought for a long time. I couldn't decide. How can you choose when every single patient has touched your life in some way? One night, though, I couldn't sleep and I started thinking about it again. I thought of Gary and I started to cry. I grieve the loss of my friend and all these years later, I remember him and his smile. I remember his voice and his way of making everyone around him feel better. He was a part of my life for almost all of my life. He was so kind to me and helped me when I was a kid. I hope in some way I was able to help him as an adult.

Gary truly lived his life and I wish he had had more time - to live and to love. He had so much to give. I was so fortunate to have him in my life and if I were writing in his yearbook today, I would say "to Gary, a friend I will never forget."

Donna Fleming, MSSW
Beverly, West Virginia

Briefly Knowing Michael

Michael didn't know he had mild hemophilia. He played on his high school football team and loved to horse around with his friends. He led a very "normal" life which included getting an occasional bruise now and then. I don't think he gave hemophilia a second thought. In fact, in his younger years, he probably didn't even know what it was.

Michael was diagnosed with mild hemophilia at age 16 when he had surgery to correct a broken nose. Later that year, after getting his driver's license, he was hit by a drunk driver and suffered several broken ribs which, in turn, ruptured his spleen. During the surgery to repair his spleen he received clotting factor and lots of cryoprecipitate. It was 1983, and unknown to the doctors who were treating him, the blood products were contaminated with HIV. Michael contracted the HIV virus. Over the next seven years his health slowly declined. He succumbed to AIDS in April, 1990. He was 23 years old.

Michael was the first person with hemophilia and HIV that I met when I started my job with the Hemophilia Council of California. I made a home visit and was very nervous since I didn't yet know much about hemophilia. I knew more about HIV since my previous job had been providing HIV test results to patients. As it turned out, Michael was relatively new in his knowledge of his own hemophilia, but sadly, he had come to know quite a bit about HIV. These were the years when the anti-viral treatments (AZT, ddI) were very toxic and not nearly as effective in curbing infections as the medications that are used routinely today. Looking back, Michael was as much a victim of bad timing and bad luck as anyone I've known who had a bleeding disorder and HIV.

Being new in my job and not sure what to talk with him about, we somehow landed on a subject he and his mom cared for deeply. Popular music. One thing I did know about young men from both personal experience and previous jobs, was that "talking about their feelings" was often not their favorite pastime. So we found ways to use music as some kind of common ground or parallel language. The Beatles and the Pretenders were frequent subjects. Dissecting the lyrics to "Nowhere Man" or raving about our mutual fascination with the guitar solo on the Pretender's song "Kid" became part of our lexicon. Our mutual comfort with the language of music slowly opened the doors for deeper conversations to form and flourish.

Michael spent a fair amount of time in the hospital during the last year of his life. We continued our talks at his bedside. I had the privilege of getting to know a very strong and kind young man who had some dreams that would never be realized. The gifts he gave to those of us who knew him were many. His legacy has continued on for years after his death.

One of the greatest gifts that Michael gave to me was the opportunity to know his mother, Bonnie Joy. Michael was her only child, and when he passed away, she was emotionally devastated by the loss. I made a number of home visits over the ensuing months to spend time with Bonnie Joy, to sit and listen to her tell stories, or to let her softly cry. Sometimes we simply sat in silence while she missed her wonderful son. In hindsight, I slowly became aware of the astounding grace that she showed to her family, her friends, and the medical providers as she bravely grieved her son's death. She has certainly taught me more about the art of grieving than anyone I have ever known.

Years later when Michael would have turned thirty, in November, 1997, Bonnie Joy sent out fancy invitations asking about sixty people to attend a "30th birthday party" in his honor. I received an invitation at my office and was initially taken aback. Was Bonnie Joy really throwing her deceased son a birthday party? Was she sure this was a good idea?

It turned out to be one of the most healing activities in which I have ever participated. Almost everyone who was invited attended. There was lots of good food and lively conversation. After a few hours of spirited chatter, the guests were summoned to the kitchen where a select group of people read something they had prepared. They shared a poem or a prayer; even a funny story. A number of others chimed in with sweet anecdotal stories about Michael. His best friend was there, as was the chaplain who had ministered to him in the last months of his life. They all came to laugh and to cry and to celebrate, with his mother, Michael's short but wonderful life. I became aware of what a powerful gift I had been given when I met this young man and his mom. Lessons about patience, love, perseverance, humor, and compassion were there for the taking every time I visited their home. These lessons continued for years after Michael's life ended. I still see Bonnie Joy from time to time. She and her son taught me much about life and death, grief and loss, tragedy and redemption. I will always be very thankful to both of them.

Dana Francis, MSW
San Francisco, California

Not Quite What I Was Planning

Not Quite What I Was Planning was a 2008 *New York Times* bestseller. The title was a six-word memoir of true life stories that were written by writers "famous and obscure". The stories were concise but moving, fascinating, and occasionally humorous. As social workers, we have been given the special privilege to intersect with families at critical times in their lives. To select six-word life stories would be impossible and impractical; however, I concur that my 33-year journey with the families of individuals with bleeding disorders is *Not Quite What I Was Planning*. In fact, it is far more meaningful and significant than I could have ever imagined. It is a journey which enabled me to participate in many joyful moments, e.g., attending graduations, weddings, band concerts, or heartrending moments in writing eulogies, attending funerals, or making a quilt for a youth who died of AIDS through contaminated blood transfusions. These moments have enlarged and deepened my life experience.

There were many, many "learning moments" etched in my memories, making it difficult to choose which story or stories to share. However, two unique ones come to mind. One is inspired by recent interests in trauma prevention and treatment and the other is the sheer joy of seeing the "medical world" through the eyes of a child. Both encounters opened my eyes to seeing life from two very different perspectives.

The first story is from a by-gone era, yet is very relevant to current national mental health concerns. The story took place in the mid-1980s, when a father who had never accompanied his son to the hemophilia clinic, made an appointment himself to bring his son. He wanted to learn more about his son's bleeding disorder and, more specifically, to find out about some new tests the medical staff recommended that his son have. I was very excited about his wish to learn more about hemophilia. Happily,

I armed myself with lots of pamphlets, insurance information, and helpful resources. I thought I was well prepared to utilize this opportunity to encourage and praise this father's involvement in his son's care.

I entered the examination room following the medical team members' visit. With an upbeat voice, I introduced myself. What ensued was something I did not anticipate. This father started to shout at me, gesturing vigorously, and ordering me to "get out of the room." The medical team, who had just left the room, looked as bewildered as I was, asking what happened. I was, of course, quite embarrassed and confused. It was only later, much later the following day when the child's mother called to apologize and told us that the father had a flashback to his Vietnam War experience. He was a veteran with memories that he didn't talk much about, except during his unpredictable flashbacks. When he saw me, an Asian, he suddenly imagined he was being attacked by the Vietcong. Weeks later when I saw this father in the clinic again, he gave permission for me to speak to him. I learned to tolerate not knowing if I could offer any help or support, but only to listen quietly to needs that were not what I thought they should be. I learned patience for when, and if, he would feel safe enough to share.

Today, with the political climate in the Middle East, and thousands of returning veterans with diagnosed or undiagnosed PTSD or brain injuries, my experience with this father, a returning traumatized veteran, will most likely be repeated. I hope HTC's with increasing numbers of medical staff and team members from the Middle East or other foreign countries will be better prepared and trained to recognize and handle similar encounters.

The second story I would like to share was about a seven year old child, "Johnny", (not his real name). Johnny and his family arrived at the hospital on a late Saturday afternoon. They came to participate in one of our annual clinic family outings. That day, we were to take a group trip to see a professional soccer game. They came quite early, before most of the other families' arrived. Johnny and his siblings were running outside the hospital main entrance; their mother was seated in the lobby. I arrived with food delivery service, pushing carts with boxed meals. Johnny spotted me and he ran back into the lobby quickly to tell his mother. I heard him shouting loudly to her, "She is here. I found her." His mother said, "Who is here? Who are you talking about?" He responded, much to my surprise, "You know, you know..... that doctor with the smallest feet!!!" I burst into laughter! How refreshing and delightful to see from the eyes of a child. It didn't seem to matter to him what professional category each team member represented. He had his own value system and way of organizing his world of experiences. Furthermore, our lower extremities are closer to his range of vision and observation, especially if we stand as we communicate with the parents while the child looks up at us. It reminds us of how we should position our body and our height as we talk to the children, on their eye level.

Every patient and their family, story by story, each is unique and extraordinary. What a privilege it is that they share their stories with us. Their stories may not be quite what we were planning to hear, but they are far more meaningful and significant than we could have ever imagined. As we patiently listen, learn, and grow, all our lives are better for it.

Elizabeth Fung, PhD., LCSW
Chicago, Illinois

"Douger": Miracle Boy/Miracle Man

My journey into the world of bleeding disorders began on a hot, sunny day in July 1989. I was interviewing for the position of Medical Social Worker at the Hemophilia Treatment Center in Peoria, IL. At that time, my knowledge of bleeding disorders was minimal. My only experience with HIV had been working with a patient (in a small rural community hospital) whose life was shrouded in secrecy and shame because of his HIV+ status. Although the Medical Director emphasized I would be working closely with her and with patients who were HIV+, little did I know that one of the first patients I would meet would be this precocious 4 year old boy named Douglas who I immediately nicknamed "Douger" (I still call him that!). I did not count on him capturing my heart (what about those boundary issues – what are the boundaries with a 4 year old?).

The life of the young man I call "miracle boy/miracle man" began with his birth on January 28, 1985, at Travis Air Force Base in California, where his biological father was in the military. Unfortunately, Douger had a brain bleed during birth and received whole blood. He was then diagnosed as having severe Factor VIII deficiency and received factor several times thereafter. His home/social environment was chaotic (especially with the recent birth of a daughter) and his mother, in particular, felt overwhelmed with his medical needs. At age 14 months Douger's parents asked his mother's uncle and aunt to care for him in a small community in central IL. At age 17 months, he experienced a bleed requiring treatment. His mother (parents were now divorced) refused to come to IL to give permission for treatment, so the state department of children and family services was contacted. Douger's aunt and uncle then became his foster parents. At this time, Douger was found to be HIV+ from having received contaminated factor sometime between his birth and 17 months of age. As I learned this history from his foster mom, I remember feeling this was a child "born too soon," since a few months later, screening of all blood became mandatory. He remained in foster care with his aunt and uncle until he was almost 5, at which time they adopted him (and his 4 y/o sister for whom they had also been caring).

From the very beginning, Douger amazed me with his intelligence and verbal skills. He had an unbelievable understanding (for a child of his age) of his hemophilia and HIV+ diagnoses. I always attributed a great deal of that knowledge/understanding to the openness with which his adopted mom talked with him. I remember once during a clinic visit when he was very young, his mom shared that on the way to clinic Douger had asked her if he was going to die. She very calmly and directly began a discussion with him (at his level of understanding) on the subject of death –WOW! Douger seemed quite satisfied with his mom's explanation. I was not at all sure that I could have handled that question so well!

At the young age of 6, Douger and his mother appeared on the Phil Donahue Show, sharing their family's experience living with HIV, especially in a conservative, small Midwestern town. From that time forward, he became a fantastic educator/role model. His mother says he even educated his friends not to touch him if he got hurt when they were playing if he was bleeding. His story appeared in local newspapers, and he and his mother participated in many activities/events to raise awareness, as well as money, for AIDS research.

Although he responded well to his HIV treatment, on his 7th birthday, Douger was diagnosed with Burkett's Lymphoma (at that time, there were only 3 others in the country with the diagnosis, only one being a child and the other two deceased). He was flown by life flight helicopter to St. Jude Children's Hospital in Memphis where he spent two months, then received 14 months of follow-up treatment at the local St. Jude affiliate in Peoria, IL. I remember being with Douger and his mother as they boarded the helicopter and thinking I would never see this child alive again. I was filled with extreme sadness and grief. I also recall many telephone conversations with his mother crying and asking me if she had "done the right thing" as the treatments at St. Jude were excruciating for him. As I listened to his mother's tearful voice, I felt so helpless and inadequate. As a mother, I could simply not imagine having to make the decision to allow treatment that offered no absolute guarantee of success. At one point during the treatment, his mother came home to purchase a casket and a cemetery plot. Selfishly, I was thankful she did not ask me to go with her (as other parents had previously asked me to help plan their child's funeral).

Today at age 28, Douger is doing well physically and emotionally. His Burkett's Lymphoma has been in remission for many years, and his HIV is being managed. He is in a stable relationship and employed as an assistant manager of a retail store. Douger remains close to his family and even gave his old social worker a big hug during the Christmas season when he recognized me in a store. When I spoke with him recently on the phone about writing "his story", he laughed and told me to "write a tall tale". I told him his life was a "tall tale"! He then said maybe he could be considered a miracle since he was still alive and doing well. I believe Douger is a wonderful example of not only modern medicine, but more importantly, the miracle of hope, faith, and love! I am truly thankful my heart was indeed captured by that precocious 4 year old. I learned so many life lessons from Douger and his mom and will be forever grateful to know them.

Linda Gammage, MSW, LCSW
Peoria, Illinois

Tomorrow's Another Day

With a knock at my office door, he filled the doorway. Tall and solid, he resembled a linebacker for the New England Patriots. But then he smiled and he filled the room with his warmth. That was my first meeting with Jim, a man with mild hemophilia A, who had stopped in to meet me, the new social worker.

When I joined the New England Hemophilia Center in 1990, the staff had already experienced what turned out to be the worst of the HIV epidemic. The nation had lost many people with hemophilia and our staff and patients were dealing physically and emotionally with the repercussions.

I often think of Jim, who had considered himself so lucky to have evaded contracting HIV, only to discover years later that he had Hepatitis C, a battle that he was not destined to win.

Through the years, I had the pleasure of getting to know Jim well through his medical visits and many phone calls. He was a gregarious, outgoing man who smiled quickly and joked even more easily. His sense of humor was his trademark and he wore it well. His concern was for others first – his family, friends, and colleagues. Somehow, he seemed to always maintain a positive outlook. After all, "Tomorrow's another day!" he would proclaim to me. And indeed, this became his mantra as he sought to live life to its fullest. He was never happier than when he could give something to others, whether it was a smile, a laugh, or an offer of assistance. Could he help me with anything? I was so touched when he would ask me that.

Jim worked hard to provide for his family, his loving wife and brilliant middle school-aged son. So when he was laid off from his job as a salesperson from a large corporation where he had worked for two decades, he was greatly affected. We talked often as Jim tackled the issues head on and plotted courses of action. He frequently ended his conversations with "Tomorrow's another day!" signaling his determination to find hope and opportunities wherever they may reside.

While going through his layoff, Jim also enrolled in treatment for his Hepatitis C. He had the courage to go through treatment even when the side effects were debilitating. But Jim never let the emotional effects of his layoff or the physical effects of his liver disease and treatment get him down for very long. Tomorrow would always be another day for him – a day that would perhaps offer another chance to find a job, to be cured, to feel better, to be happier or, more importantly, to make someone else happy.

When Jim found out he had developed liver cancer, he followed the path he had come to know so well. He faced it, dealt with it and gathered his resources for the fight. He went through the grueling process of tests, paperwork, and research to get on the transplant list in the Boston area. He was determined to find hope for himself and his family. Jim took control as he hoped for the best but prepared for the worst. He got his affairs in order. When the tumors became too big for transplant consideration, Jim showed his tenacity and still did not give up.

Unfortunately, tomorrow did not bring a cure and Jim's fight eventually ended in the hospital where he was surrounded by his family and friends. After his death, the memory of Jim's life brought inspiration to his family and those of us who were fortunate enough to know him. His concerns were always beyond himself toward a better tomorrow for others. In the end, Jim taught us to seek hope and opportunities to cope with life's obstacles because, after all, "Tomorrow's another day!"

Peg Geary, MA, MBA, MPH, LCSW, CCM
Worcester, Massachusetts

Courageous Journey

First and foremost, having compassion should be an attribute of any effective social worker, along with a sense of realism. We can't save the world, but having the belief that people really want to establish a better life for themselves gives me the strength and desire to go that extra mile. Thus, having this kind of passion protects me from burnout! I have always believed my career choice would lead me down a path that enables me to advocate for others. As a freshman at the University of Georgia, embarking on my first sociology class, I realized that the field of social work was my lifelong dream! Harvey MacKay once said, "Find something you love to do and you'll never work a day in your life." I concur!

My journey as a social worker began in January, 2000. I was truly blessed when I joined the adult hemophilia team at the Medical College of Georgia (presently known as Georgia Health Sciences University) in Augusta, Georgia. Hemophilia was unknown to me but I remembered Ryan White's tragic ordeal. Dr. Charles L. Lutcher was one of the pioneers instrumental in establishing our treatment center. Bridget Schausten, RN, was the nurse, and I was their student. They are both extraordinary teachers, and because of them, I would like to believe that I became well versed in bleeding disorders! Hemophilia of Georgia, Inc., is an amazing chapter and the common denominator between the chapter and our HTC is providing dedicated service to our bleeding disorders community.

All of my patients have a coping mechanism that provides them with strength to cope with the hand that they were dealt. Although when I think of strength and courage, Jerry (fictitious name) comes to mind.

Several years ago, Jerry, a man with severe hemophilia, HIV, and Hepatitis C, took himself off disability and found full-time employment. He has a loving, supportive family, a caring heart, and a very cheerful demeanor! He enjoys travel and gatherings with family and friends; he is living his life to the fullest! I have asked him to apply to be a camp counselor at Hemophilia of Georgia's Camp Wannaklot and he has promised to do so whenever time permits. He has a small child who is involved in several activities. Jerry and his wife are "hands-on" parents. Jerry does not let his disease beat him, but rather uses the strength it has created in him to touch others.

To further demonstrate Jerry's inspirational example, he mentored patients in the "Buddy Link", a mentoring program we held jointly with our pediatric hemophilia clinic. Valerie Crenshaw, RN, who is the pediatric hemophilia nurse, informed me that he did a fantastic job!

On a personal note, in 2006, when I was away from the office after surgery, Jerry retrieved what I had thought was my unlisted number from our city phone directory. He called because he was concerned about me. I assured him I was just fine! I admire the fact that Jerry is not wallowing in self-pity and is looking toward the future! He is doing well, and I am looking forward to our continuous journey!

Chartara Y. Gilchrist, BA
Augusta, Georgia

Collision

I had just started in the world of hemophilia and HIV/AIDS as a brand spankin' new social worker, the dust not yet even settled on my Master's degree. My job was funded by grants from the Centers for Disease Control to conduct research and develop programming for partners/wives of men with hemophilia and HIV. Without knowing it at that time, my life was on a direct (and delightful) collision course with Lisa.

Lisa started as my client, became my co-worker, ended as my best friend, and was the Godmother of my only daughter. How is THAT for one helluva' collision course? She was, and still is, one ballsy broad, raised by a truck driver and a feminist, with the largest heart this side of the Canadian border. Lisa continues to teach me to live fearlessly.

Lisa was the partner of Ron, who was seriously ill by the time I met them. While they were engaged, like many, they decided not to get married so Ron could maintain his healthcare coverage. I met Lisa before Ron died. I met her when she had not yet become public about her own HIV diagnosis. Always the strong one, she held the pain and sorrows of the entire world on her tiny size 2 shoulders. She had lost her parents when she was very young. She took care of an older autistic sister most of her life. Lisa had been supporting herself since the age of 15. And now, as an HIV positive woman, her priority was taking care of Ron.

Lisa did what all partners do. She listened to him, laughed with him, and enjoyed his Blues music. She bathed him, cleaned up his vomit, administered his medication, drove him to the doctor's office, and cooked for him. This was part of the package known as "love." There was never a question of leaving, even though Ron was a healthy man when they met. Ron died on Christmas Eve. He wanted so desperately to hang on until Christmas. But hanging on was a struggle. Lisa gave him permission to leave if he felt ready. She gave him permission to have peace and to leave lovingly, not with struggle and resistance.

Lisa is my teacher. She gave me permission to feel pain and to be vulnerable. She taught me that vulnerability and pain are on one side, and joy, beauty, and love are on the other. She taught me that if you just dive into that pain, experience it fully, and stay awake through the whole experience, then this amazing thing happens. You stay awake for the beauty, the joy, and the love as well.

In the years I have known Lisa I have seen people treat her like dirt. Her supposed friends, after discovering she was HIV positive, would not use her toilet. People whom she considered "family" later rejected her. Lisa not only lost the love of her life to AIDS, but also dozens of dear, beautiful friends. When the pharmaceutical settlement became final, a few people who were close to her betrayed her love. (Oh, money can bring out ugly behavior in otherwise decent people!). The painful events are too numerous to name. Needless to say, I have seen Lisa cry in pain. When the pain is so raw that it sears into your bones, your body buckles up under you. Yes, I have seen her roll into a fetal position, sobbing uncontrollably.

What is amazing about this woman are her transformative qualities. You would think that these painful experiences would render Lisa a bitter human being, but this could not be further from the truth. She took each and every moment of pain and transformed them into forgiveness and love. I guess there comes a time when you decide to either shut down and close up, or learn how to open your heart even more. This is the great lesson I have learned from Lisa. Don't close down. Yes, it is so tempting to close, to protect yourself, to move away. But keep that heart open—forgive, let go, and release—and lo and behold, the joy in your life is more bountiful than before. Lisa taught me there is nothing to be afraid of. It really does take more courage to keep the heart open and remain fully awake, because you feel all the pain. But as I have learned from Lisa, there is nothing worth closing the heart for.

I can say with all honesty there is no one who has made me laugh more than Lisa. She is an example of how one can embrace life and live it fully. Lisa takes great pleasure in cooking, reading, and music. If you want to know how to dig through the darkness and the dirt to reach the sunlight (and enjoy the heck out of that sun!), then spend a day with Lisa. It will be more educational than any class you could possibly take.

When I met Lisa, I was young and new at the whole social worker gig. I was scared and did not know how I would handle seeing clients during some of the most painful times of their lives. Step by step, I learned how to be a better social worker. The gift I received from Lisa was more universal. Lisa taught me how to be a human being.

Isabel Lin Guzman, MSW, JD
Chapel Hill, North Carolina

He Touches Lives Despite Adversity

Rick Lopez, my dear friend and former colleague, is an exceptional human being who has inspired me. He has also touched my heart in countless ways.

Rick and I met while serving on the NHF Multicultural Working Group in the late 1990's. Rick wasn't one to complain or express negativity or pessimism. His entire focus was to serve the hemophilia population, to make decisions that were in the best interest of the bleeding disorders community, and to educate clinicians on multicultural issues. His heart was always in the right place.

Rick was employed by the Hemophilia Treatment Center at Children's Hospital of Los Angeles. It is unclear what his position was, but my understanding is he had multiple responsibilities. According to his mother, Rick worked "24/7 helping others outside the hospital." Often times, his parents were unaware that he had extended himself to others until those who received his help would approach him simply to express gratitude for providing assistance, education, and/or hope.

Rick was diagnosed with hemophilia as an infant in 1960 and with HIV in 1986. He was born into a family with four other relatives who had hemophilia. He learned firsthand through these courageous relatives about hemophilia. He learned of the pain they endured, the type of treatment they received, and the challenges each one faced. Observing and being around these relatives gave Rick valuable insight, knowledge, and wisdom that would later shape his perceptions, attitudes, and coping abilities. Furthermore, it would enable him to live his life with optimism, faith, and courage as his challenges unfolded. Rick's attitude regarding hemophilia was that it was just "something that came with the territory." He has not allowed fear to take control of his life nor does he feel bitterness. His insurmountable faith holds hope for the future. His goals have been to maintain a healthy lifestyle with a life purpose of helping others.

Anti retro viral medications have been the standard form of treatment for HIV. The initial HIV medication Rick was on was not user friendly and often caused side effects that were unbearable. He tried diligently to take his HIV medications as directed, but would become extremely ill. The side effects left him bedridden, with no appetite, and extremely weak from vomiting day in and day out. Through the help of a good friend, Rick was referred to another HIV specialist who revamped his HIV medications. Unfortunately, before the new medications could help control the virus, Rick had been having mini seizures that eventually progressed to a massive seizure. Multiple physicians were involved in Rick's medical care and were confused about his diagnosis. Since he had symptoms of Progressive Multi-Focal Lymphoma (PML), his HIV doctor diagnosed him with PML and started him on seizure medication. After seizure medications were initiated, the seizures stopped. The occurrence of developing PML was considered rare because his viral count was higher than those who typically develop this medical condition.

With PML, multiple areas of the brain can be affected. Rick's speech was seriously affected. He is unable to communicate verbally. He currently communicates with a spelling board or by putting both thumbs up for yes, ok, or to demonstrate some form of happiness. Thumbs down indicates a dislike of some sort. Because Rick loves to eat, Dora, his mother, experiments with different recipes. She humorously mentioned how he will occasionally give her meal a "thumbs down" critique. She now knows which recipes not to repeat.

Rick was left paralyzed on the right side of his body. Due to having an imbalance while attempting to walk, he is confined to a wheel chair. With love and support, his family helps him navigate his wheelchair and assists in helping him get in and out of it. This routine has become a way of life for Rick and his family with no complaints or regrets.

Despite being physically incapacitated, Rick has not been deterred from living a full and abundant life. His intelligence, cognitive abilities, and sense of humor have remained intact. He returned to college and received a degree in Cultural Anthropology and graduated with honors; Summa Cum Laude. He maintains a busy schedule going on day trips, attending social gatherings, and looking forward to fundraising and cultural events. He also enjoys hanging out with family and friends, and accepting social invitations from those he has helped along his journey. He has a passion for learning about the Native American population. Watching educational channels that address the cultural and historical accounts of the indigenous tribes is an enjoyable pastime. Because writing is difficult for Rick, he writes short key words in his journal to refresh his memory about what he has learned from these educational documentaries and stories.

Rick is extremely blessed to have such an attentive, caring, loving, and nurturing family. Dora and Dick, his parents, are his primary and dedicated caretakers. His parents treat him with normalcy and kindness, and they are very conscientious about his medical needs. Dora describes Rick as very patient, never expressing bitterness about his health, and easy to take care of. Anne Marie, his sister, is also loving and caring and brings laughter, joy, and amusement to their relationship. I like to refer to Anne Marie as Rick's partner in crime!

It is with great respect that I honor Rick's immediate and extended family for teaching him the skills necessary to be a survivor. They have encouraged him to maintain a healthy outlook on life. Because of their extraordinary support and unconditional love, Rick is capable of going forward in his life with gratitude and the ability to genuinely love others. He appears to have a continual zest for life without regret!

Rick's ability to cope so well has also been due to the significant influence and support he has received from his religious beliefs, support from specific priests, and from the schooling he received from St. Joseph Elementary and Damien High School. His faith is insurmountable and he truly believes his faith will continue to help him in the future. As the saying goes, "it takes a village" to raise a person along life's journey. This indeed holds true because Rick credits many individuals with contributing to his well-being. These include friends, co-workers, teachers, and "even some I have not met but who have helped me in some way."

According to Rick, his spiritual identity of "who I have been, who I am, and who I will be," has its roots in the family he has known, starting with grandparents, parents, his sister, aunts, and uncles. In one way or another, his family has generously given back to the community through donating their time, special talents, and resources to make this world a better place.

Rick has learned to be a genuine and selfless humanitarian due to the role modeling his family has demonstrated, but mostly by his tremendous and personal desire to help those in need. On a spiritual level, helping others is his purpose. He began making charitable contributions long before he became ill. His goodwill has been spread through various means: monetary donations, emotional support, and education. Rick looks forward to attending fund raising events because they allow him other opportunities to help someone, or to support a cause. In fact, years ago, Rick donated funds to build a one room home for a family in Mexico. Besides monetary contributions, Rick has paved a road of hope for the forgotten individuals who feel isolated, afraid, and uncertain about their future. He donates without expecting anything in return and without expecting recognition (his charitable work was relayed to me by his mother).

While serving on the Multicultural Working Group with Rick, I quickly took notice of his kindness and his intelligence. I was in awe of how humble he was. He rarely shared the trials and tribulations of his life with me because that isn't who he is. After one of our meetings, I will always remember with fondness the wonderful time we had together drinking Prickly Pear martinis, getting further acquainted, and sharing memorable stories about ourselves. Years later, our friendship resumed and despite the distance between us, we have somehow managed to stay in touch.

I had the opportunity to visit Rick on one occasion while I was in California. Our visit was very endearing and wonderful. During the visit his family shared stories about Rick's current medical condition. They also showed me newspaper articles of Rick's achievements. We later went to a restaurant and while enjoying lunch, Anne Marie told these absolutely humorous stories that brought continual laughter and joy. It was an unforgettable experience to hear Rick laugh and to observe the joy, happiness, and fun he was experiencing.

I'm truly blessed to have Rick in my life! He has inspired me to be a better person, to continue my work with the hemophilia population with passion and compassion, and to never give up when I'm faced with my own challenges. Through our special friendship and from knowing who Rick is, I've learned the meaning of strength, tremendous courage, resilience, determination, kindness, and generosity. I've also learned the spirit of being true to oneself regardless of one's circumstances.

With gratitude, I'm happy and honored to have Rick as my friend and my teacher! In conclusion, the following passage applies to Rick: "To the World, you may be one person, but to one person, you are the World!"

Margaret Halona, MSW, LMSW
Albuquerque, New Mexico

Where Do I Begin?

I have been the social worker at an HTC since October, 1989, so I have met many individuals and families over the years and have seen the world of hemophilia go through many changes. In thinking about who might have had the most impact on me as a social worker, it is difficult to pick one individual, as each person/family has had their unique impact. Let me share some of my thoughts about those I have encountered.

I first have to share about another social worker, Donna, who I met early on in my career at the HTC. She was from the same region and we would see each other at meetings. Donna has a social worker's heart. She was always interested in the welfare of her patients and families with whom she worked and wanted what was best for them. She helped me "survive" my first hemophilia summer camp experience which was before I had been at the HTC a year. I was still learning about hemophilia and the community and she was such a great role model and an inspiration for me. She related so well to the campers and staff, had loads of energy, and knew when to be serious but also knew how to have lots of fun. She instilled a love for camp in me. Thank you, Donna.

Where do I begin? Our center sees both children and adults so I've had the privilege to meet people at different stages in their lives. I think of Mike who moved here from another part of the country with his wife and who was always amazed that he was alive in his 40's. He had been told he would never live past his teen years because he had severe hemophilia. He was co-infected with HIV and HCV. He had had three knee replacements. He was smart, funny, and he worked hard. The last few years were a challenge for him and he struggled, but he left an imprint on this world.

There is Dennis who was in his thirties with severe hemophilia, HIV, and HCV. He was a country boy who found a woman (and her two children) whom he loved dearly. He was a hard worker and worked as long as he could. He also liked to fish and hunt and would take his nephew out when he had time off. One of his last jobs was near the hospital so sometimes he would stop by and we would talk. He knew he might not live a long life but was trying to live a full life and also making plans for his family for when he was no longer here. I had the opportunity to visit him in his home near the end of his life and even when he was in pain he had a positive attitude and was always thinking of his family.

Shawn was a young man I knew from the time he was camp age. He had severe hemophilia, HIV, and HCV. But that did not matter in how he approached life. He completed high school, started working, and remained a dedicated and hard working person until the very end of his life which was last year (2012), when he was in his mid-thirties. He had hoped a liver transplant would work, but it didn't, unfortunately. I always looked forward to Shawn coming to clinic. When he was young, one or both of his parents would accompany him, but as soon as he was old enough he came on his own. His parents instilled in him the importance of being responsible which led to his strong work ethic, and his strong faith. I knew he had many friends he kept up with from high school as well as those from his church. Not until his funeral, though, did I see the impact that his life had had on so many people. I never heard him say anything negative about anyone, and he loved his family. Shawn always kept a sense of humor and his high moral standards. He was a joy to be around.

Each of the above individuals was different. What I learned from them was about being true to yourself, having resiliency, positive thinking, a strong work ethic, the importance of family and friends, and having a sense of humor. These qualities help us get through the toughest of times. They also taught me to enjoy each day, make the most of that day, and to slow down, take a deep breath, and use all your senses to take everything in. They reinforced that what is important in life is your faith, your family, and your friends.

It has been an interesting journey being the HTC social worker. There have been so many changes in hemophilia care. The men I've already mentioned were ones who had to cope with so many things whereas the younger children/teens don't have as many barriers. Yes, it is still an expensive medical condition. And yes, there are many emotions that parents experience when they learn their child has hemophilia, but the individual with hemophilia can participate in activities that those in previous generations were unable to do. There is preventive treatment for joint bleeds which is such a blessing. Because the new factor replacement is not a blood product, there are fewer concerns about blood borne diseases.

It has been both a privilege, and at times a challenge, being a social worker within the hemophilia community, but one that I would not trade. I have seen so many children grow up to be adults with their own families. There are so many other examples that could be shared of stories such as the young man with severe hemophilia who is a doctor, one who is in dental school, one who works in the biogenetics industry, and the many who have wives, parents, and friends who are there for them. I have also had the privilege to meet so many colleagues with dedication not only to the profession of social work, but to the individuals within the hemophilia and bleeding disorders community. I am honored to call many of them my friends. I have been blessed.

Mavis Harrop, MSSW, LCSW
Nashville, Tennessee

The Last Best Minute

Coming straight out of graduate school into the newly formed position of Hemophilia Social Worker at Cook County Hospital (now called Stroger Hospital of Cook County) threw me into cultural shock. It wasn't the first time I had gone through something like that. There had been the time in college when I spent the spring trimester in Spain. Coping with cultural shock was a deliberate part of the educational experience, back before the time of smart phones with translation help, when going to a Spanish-speaking country meant actually having to converse in Spanish, wretched as my conversational Spanish was. I remember feeling I was never entirely sure what people were saying. Then at night or during the long Spanish siestas in the afternoon, I would sleep and dream. In my dreams I would be listening to Spaniards talking in classrooms, bars, and stores, with me still not quite comprehending. I felt the linguistic centers in my brain working overtime, trying to put it all together.

I persevered and gained enough capacity to dare to apply to a job that required Spanish-language ability. The County had battled with the federal government to gain recognition as a Pediatric and Adult Hemophilia Treatment Center (HTC) in order to qualify for the grants that paid for the social work position. Because the job was grant-funded and required bilingual skills, I was the only applicant. I didn't know anything about hemophilia, and I understood the world of the poor only a little, despite having some experience in social services when I worked for two years at a food bank between undergraduate and graduate school. It was the time of the AIDS crisis in the hemophilia world. I felt like I would have the opportunity to make a difference in peoples' lives through traditional social work interactions. And, most pragmatically, I had to make a living and pay off my student loans.

One of the great benefits of being the first person in a new position is you don't have any predecessor to whom you will be ranked and compared. In fact, very little is fixed, there is room to improvise. That may seem exciting, but I rarely experienced it that way in the beginning. I introduced myself to patients, offered to help, read up on hemophilia, and had long conversations with a staff person at the local chapter (then called the Hemophilia Foundation of Illinois) who had worked at the County Hospital earlier in his career. The patients weren't responding to me the way I had anticipated and when I became frustrated, I retreated into studying and felt justified doing so. I had been hired before I even had the opportunity to sit for the exam to become a basic Licensed Social Worker, but there was one coming up in a few months and the rules were clear. I had to pass that exam or I would be fired.

Studying for the exam was merely the beginning of my on-the-job learning. The County managed to win recognition as an HTC because of the number of patients with bleeding disorders being treated, but we were not functioning as a "normal" HTC. For one thing there had never been any staff to do follow-up between hematology clinic visits or after ER visits and inpatient stays. After a while I realized "I'm it. I'm the person who is going to have to figure out a way to make us into something more like a 'normal' HTC." I felt more than a little daunted. I went through a period of insomnia. It didn't help that I also wanted to have some more typical warm and fuzzy social work-style relationships with the patients, and the patients were not used to having anyone trying to work with them like that. I had the right background in terms of degrees and language skills, and even a certificate in health administration that I had earned along with my MSW, but the difference between theory and practice seemed as wide as the ocean. I remember one helpful thing that one of the physicians who helped to get me hired said to me, and it went like this: "Don't get frustrated about being frustrated. You are getting paid to be frustrated."

Passing that licensing test gave me some sense of accomplishment in that first difficult year. But it was the compensation offered via a class action suit against the manufacturers of the anti-hemophilia product (that had infected many of the patients with HIV) that finally helped me get some ground under my feet. At last I had a clear task that would allow me to engage with the patients. In 1992, there were few proven treatments for HIV disease and there would not be any developed for several years. Many of the patients had not even been tested. The possibility of receiving $100,000 in compensation from the class action lawsuit gave patients an incentive to find out their HIV status, and having an accurate count of HIV infected patients was something the federal government wanted. It was a "normal" HTC thing to have.

Several years before I came to the County, there had been a system whereby adults with active bleeds had been able to come to the Coagulation Laboratory to receive anti-hemophilia factor. It was a somewhat informal system, discontinued understandably because it was disruptive to the work of the lab, and because it did not have the formal safeguards of an emergency room in case a patient had an allergic reaction, for example, and went into life-threatening anaphylactic shock. Of course, there had never been even a single case of anaphylactic shock in the ten years or so that hemophilia patients had been receiving anti-hemophilia product in what we called "the Coag Lab." All that notwithstanding, it was a system whose time was over. The problem was the patients loved getting their factor in the coag lab, and they hated going to the emergency room. The switch turned what had been a one-hour process into a four-to-ten-hour one. Listening to the complaints about the long wait in the ER gave me the conviction I needed to find ways to give almost every patient the opportunity to get their routine bleeds treated at home. Figuring out home care (we had only a few pediatric patients using it when I arrived in 1992) became a second focus of my attempts to create a "normal" HTC.

The coag lab also held precious records that became very important to the patients as they stepped forward to get tested for HIV and apply for compensation if the test was positive. To qualify for compensation, patients had to demonstrate both a positive HIV status and a medical record that proved they had received factor during the years when contaminated factor was prevalent. Patients began to call me when they discovered that the official medical records did not contain the crucial proof they needed. I poked around the coag lab and the office of the hematology nurse until I was certain I had gathered what turned out to be extremely valuable records. I became a detective, sorting through old documents to find what was, in some cases, the only proof that would allow a man with hemophilia and HIV to get his financial compensation. I redoubled my efforts to contact every patient for whom I had a phone number, asking them to please be sure of their HIV status. I remember talking to a middle-aged patient I'll call "Jack." Jack told me he was "pretty sure" he had tested negative for HIV. As he was a patient with very mild hemophilia who rarely bled, and who rarely needed factor, I accepted his answer and asked him to stay in touch.

Jack did stay in touch. He called me about ten days before the deadline for the class-action compensation and told me that he had confused the HIV test with another one, and his actual first HIV test had just come back positive. We sprang into action to meet the deadline. What I remember best about that time is all the help we received at Western Union Currency Exchange. I had always thought of currency exchanges as sleazy businesses that ripped off the poor with excessive fees. But Jack was received there warmly by a woman behind the glass enclosure who had known him for decades. She quickly and efficiently helped us get everything we needed to finish up the application and Jack received his compensation. It was the first of many last-minute collaborations we shared together

Somehow by the time the Ricky Ray Act had been passed and funded, about seven years later, I had forgotten about the close call with the class-action compensation. I was busy with all sorts of tasks related to home care, and I was the main person responsible for executing the Universal Data Collection (UDC) Program that the Centers for Disease Control required. It was a ton of work, but it also helped us to become more organized in our outpatient clinic work and gave me an impetus to recruit the help of the physical therapists in a more collaborative way. In the midst of all that, I almost forgot about Jack. Jack became the last patient I helped to get paperwork prepared for the federal government's compensation plan. There was a last minute snafu when we checked the Ricky Ray paperwork and realized Jack needed a routing number from his bank savings account. I had set up a "lunch and learn" session during the clinic time and was running back and forth from the clinic, where I was collecting UDC data, to the meeting room. Fortunately, a representative from one of the pharmaceutical companies that had sponsored our "lunch and learn" was able to use her cell phone to call Jack's bank and help him obtain the number.

Setting up that "lunch and learn" was only possible because the County managed to find money (from many sources) to open up an entirely new building for Infectious Diseases, called the Core Center. There were a few years at the beginning when the hematologist and I could set up hemophilia-only clinics and take advantage of the new clinic areas before they became filled exclusively with infectious disease patients. We obtained a new site for our hemophilia clinic later when Cook County Hospital built a new main building and renamed itself "Stroger Hospital of Cook County." I remember it was at one of our early "hemophilia-only" clinics that Jack came into the clinic to review some blood work with the hematologist. He had decided to try taking the anti-viral treatment for Hepatitis C while continuing the anti-viral treatment that had been controlling his HIV infection. The combination became dangerous. All his blood counts were crashing from the combined toxicities of the treatments. The hematologist told him to stop the hepatitis treatment immediately. He stopped in time to keep his bone marrow functioning.

During the clinic visits and the scrambling for compensation deadlines, I had the chance to get to know Jack, and my admiration for him deepened. He was one of only a few among my adult patients who managed to work the same job year after year, decade after decade, stay married to the same woman, and together with her, raise their children. He told me his goal was to work until he was 62. Then he could get regular Social Security retirement benefits and a pension from the bottling plant where he worked. He didn't know if he could make it. There was the untreated hepatitis, and the new managers of the company were the sort of people who "wouldn't let anyone tell them anything," as Jack put it. They put him into jobs he had done decades before. He contemplated just giving up the working life and going onto disability at times, but other times when he felt better, he contemplated working longer. I felt that retiring at 62 was the best thing for him, and I told him so. Then I realized I had gotten too attached to the idea of seeing him actually make it to retirement alive and able to enjoy a pension. I told him (and myself) that those decisions were up to him.

Since my first half-year of work in 1992, I have attended the funerals of my patients whenever possible. We lost many of them to AIDS of course, sometimes combined with failing livers. Then there were the patients who died from brain bleeds. For me it is a point of honor to be the person who represents the County at the funerals and demonstrates to the families that the lives of their loved ones have meant something to us. I also do it because it is a "normal" HTC thing to do. And I do it because it helps me to understand the lives of my patients better. In 2009, the long-established patients stopped dying (and there have been fewer deaths as of this writing in May, 2013), and I was forced, as never before, to help them fend off imminent homelessness because of the high unemployment of the Great Recession.

During a two-and-a-half year period when it seemed like almost every patient or family needed emergency financial assistance, I had the occasion to talk to one of Jack's many cousins. We were chatting about various family members we both knew when he mentioned Jack was going to retire in a few weeks. Then the thought occurred to me there was a three-year gap between retirement at age 62 and the start of Medicare coverage at age 65. I called Jack and explained the COBRA law and how he could pay a monthly fee to keep his health insurance. He talked to the human resources people at his company and signed up for the extension of his insurance. I saw him about half a year later at a picnic and he looked so good. Retirement suited him very well, psychologically and physically. His immune system was strong and his liver was still functioning. I told him how happy I was he had made it to retirement, and how I had hoped to see him thriving like that. He looked at me and said, "Yeah, I know you were hoping for it."

After almost 21 years in the job, I can look back on my early experience with greater understanding. I thought my academic and work experience and my good will would allow me to step into a different world than any I had known before. I had hoped I could overcome the barriers between my white, middle-class, raised-in-Montana upbringing and the lives of poor urban people, mostly African-American and Latino, who need (or choose) a County Hospital. I thought I could make the whole system function better. I thought I could do it, and I was right. It just took much longer than I expected to bring order out of chaos and to develop the close relationships I thought would happen automatically when I first became a social worker.

Now I'm also an honorary Blood Brother and I attend the meetings with the older guys with hemophilia who constitute a group founded by the local chapter. Most of them are my patients. We have the sort of relationship that guys form after many years together and many battles fought. Jack is one of the Brothers. And when I look back on our work together, and all the successful last-minute collaborations, I wonder what our last best minute together will be? I think it is necessary for us as social workers to have our fond hopes for good outcomes for our patients. We do what we can to make those outcomes more likely. Yet we need to hold on to those hopes lightly. We don't need our patients to be, or to do something for us thats not what the patient wants, or what is actually possible for them. Hoping comes from caring, but needing crosses the line into a betrayal of our role. It is not always an easy boundary to mind. But it sure is sweet when one of our fond hopes comes true.

Robert E. Johnson, MDiv, MSW, LCSW
Chicago, Illinois

His Medicine Costs Too Much

Watch the children run and play
Happy smiles, happy cries,
N'er a thought of pain or hurt
They are free to fly.

But for one who bleeds too much
He can't run, he can't play,
He must sit alone and watch
His medicine costs too much.

"Let me run and let me play
Be a child, just as they,
Give me that which sets me free."
No–your medicine costs too much.

Can you look into his eyes
Tell him why, tell him why,
Others have gold and jewels and such
But his medicine costs too much.

Can you look into his eyes
Tell him why, tell him why,
What he needs to set him free
His medicine costs too much.

Watch the children run and play
Happy smiles, happy cries
But for one who sits alone
His medicine costs too much.

Emily Czapek, MD
East Peoria, Illinois

Memories of John

I don't know when I first met John. I think it was in 2001 when he came for a comprehensive clinic, but then he left our treatment center for a while and did not come back for several years. I had come to the hospital in 1997, but didn't start in hemophilia until May of 1999. I had joined the Hemophilia Treatment Team after the charge nurse, Linda, became the new Nurse Coordinator. She asked if I was interested in joining her as part of the team (let's give credit where credit is due). I certainly was interested in adding to my repertoire, doing something different, and being part of a smaller team, so this was a perfect fit!

John was, from the outset, one of the people most willing to work with me, a newbie to the bleeding disorder community, and he taught me about hemophilia by freely responding to my questions, filling in gaps, and by sharing his experiences of growing up with a bleeding disorder. He didn't judge, and he had a pretty good sense of humor, accompanied by faith and family.

John was born in 1947 and at that time there was really no treatment. He told me that he had been diagnosed at about 6 months of age and that he had an older brother who bruised easily and had died of pneumonia a year before John was born. (I wondered if he had just started to cough up blood and the blood kept coming....but John would not know the answer to that question).

At the time I met him, he had already had ankle fusions, knee surgery, and his elbows were damaged enough to restrict his ability to infuse at times. He had HIV and Hepatitis C. Of course, both were acquired because of factor products made from tainted blood prior to the onset of purification processes. John worked in our hospital system as a lab technician and had a bachelor's degree in Medical Technology. He was on his feet a lot, which certainly was stressful on his joints. He also had 4 children; three sons and a daughter. He was walking for exercise, and his hobbies included hunting (for deer, duck, and anything else), boating, fishing, skeet shooting, writing, cooking, travel, reading, computers, classical music, and current events. Not too shabby for someone with physical disabilities including ankle joint fusions, knee problems, and elbow problems! I could not believe that he was able to figure out ways to do all of these activities by making some modifications! He was always analyzing.

When John returned to our HTC in 2004, he had stopped working and was receiving disability since he was having an increasingly difficult time being on his feet at the lab. He could remain busy by writing articles for "HemAware" and other publications, and by being active in the bleeding disorder community. John was trying to maintain his hobbies and interests in spite of his limitations. He was a fisherman, a boater, and he and a group of other men participated in a day of fishing on Lake Michigan. I heard that he had to be lifted out of the boat at the end of day. He also loved to cook and contributed recipes to our newsletter, the "Bleeder's Digest."

Over the next few years, John told me about missing school frequently as a youngster and spending long periods of time in the wards at Children's Hospital of Michigan where he received plasma or cryoprecipitate. He met some of the other folks who had hemophilia and they developed a camaraderie and friendship out of their common bond of wanting to be normal children in spite of a physical disability. Once at a dinner meeting several years ago, as he and another attendee were introducing themselves and starting to tell their stories, they both realized that they had been in the same special school together because of their bleeding disorder. They started telling the group about the teachers and the pranks they would play. They were just kids trying to be "normal."

He continued to enjoy seeing other adult men who had survived the disaster of HIV which took the lives of many of their peers in the community. Survivorship strengthened their bond and they would take time to meet, even if briefly, at any hemophilia event. At "Springfest", the annual educational and networking consumer conference sponsored by the Hemophilia Foundation of Michigan, he wanted to ensure that the young adults, for whom treatment had always been available, knew the history and issues involved in making such huge strides in hemophilia care and treatment. He wanted them to appreciate how far things had come.

Gradually, John began to have more medical problems, some of which were also complications from the medications used to treat his HIV and HCV, including kidney failure, which resulted in his need for dialysis. While this was certainly a setback, he was able to use his medical/lab knowledge to become an active participant in the process as the HTC physician and nurse practitioner/coordinator, together with the nephrology team, mulled over the best method for access. Although he could no longer work, John helped us investigate whether his factor infusion should be done before or after his dialysis, including whether the factor would get dialyzed out. I should state that John also felt he could modify his medications based upon his knowledge, so there were times that his pain medication regimens were discussed as he sought answers to some of the problematic side effects.

John developed liver failure and was placed on a couple of transplant lists. He struggled mightily when he was rejected for a liver transplant because of the reluctance of institutions to perform a transplant in someone with both kidney and liver failure. He wrote letters. He was not one to just give up!

By the time I really started working with him in 2004, he was in his mid-50's! As we gradually worked together more and more, I remember he once told me, "I never thought I'd live this long....now what do I do?" He shared with me that his parents had been told that he "wouldn't live past 10..." and "wouldn't live past 20...", then "wouldn't live past 30." Hearing this had a major impact on him and he had decided to live life fully and do whatever he could physically.

It was certainly an eye opener to hear that from someone who had survived a childhood with no treatment, to being able to have treatment, getting himself through school, and becoming a productive employee, husband, and father. It struck me that he was resilient in ways even he couldn't recognize.

We had periodically talked about this over the last few years. I asked him what he thought accounted for his ability to keep getting up every day and moving forward. For him, it was faith, family, and friends. It was just not giving in to the pain and the bleeding; he didn't think it was anything special. I certainly thought that the ability to go forward exhibited by John and my other adult patients demonstrated something special, unique, and strong.

The last couple of years of John's life were not as he wanted. He was in and out of the hospital and went to long-term acute care and then to a skilled nursing facility. One skilled nursing center agreed to take him and then refused because of his factor infusions. The case manager on the hospital floor worked hard to help place him in another skilled nursing facility which allowed his family to bring his factor into his room and administer it.

These placements were the most difficult for him because he was aware that providers in these facilities did not know a lot about hemophilia. He continued to play as active a role in his care as he could. He worked hard to educate the nursing staff about his condition and its impact, providing personal insight and education. Our HTC team also went out to meet and teach his new healthcare team. Eventually the nurses were willing and able to administer his infusions.

John did wonder why God had helped him survive so long only for him to face continually declining physical abilities. I am sure he really did not have the chance to discuss his questions with his priest to the depth that he wanted. Eventually John died of all the complications. Though expected, his death was a big blow to those of us who knew him, worked with him both in and out of the treatment center, and who loved him. While he is physically missed, he truly remains an integral part of the bleeding disorder community. The lessons he taught us so patiently will continue on.

Ellen Kachalsky, MSW, LMSW, ACSW
Detroit, Michigan

Danny

"Susan, you were in despair over his behavior and his antics." This was how Danny was remembered by one of my former colleagues. When I met Danny, he was in his thirties, and severely disabled in every way one could imagine. In addition to severe hemophilia, Hepatitis C, and HIV, he had brain damage due to early abuse by his father. He was good-hearted, fun-loving, and possessed a surprisingly high degree of social skills. However, he was learning impaired, to say the least, with an IQ of (reportedly) 75, and he never learned to read.

The comment above was provoked by Danny's blowing out his motorized scooter on one of Seattle's very steep hills. Enjoying company and always generous, he was offering tows to his friends who had wheelchairs without motors, and who struggled on the hills. He was trying to help others while enjoying himself. What could possibly go wrong? Well, things did go wrong. Danny, coached by the staff at the Puget Sound Blood Center (HTC) to ask questions, to be as independent as possible, and to articulate his needs, did just that. He kept requesting (demanding) a new motorized scooter. Need I say how expensive this was? Need I say that the State's Medicaid program did not allow replacing relatively new medical equipment? Well, let's just say that assertiveness training for Danny was definitely effective. However, his patience (never his strongest trait), was tested, and my powers of explanation were sorely tested.

This slightly hilarious and heartbreaking episode took some time to resolve as I fielded what seemed like hourly questions about the arrival of the new scooter. Danny learned he could not offer folks a tow, even in the relatively flat areas around Seattle's Pike Place Market. Eventually a replacement scooter arrived. However, more damage ensued because he would forget that his scooter was plugged in and recharging. He would start to move, forgetting about the plug, and would rip the plug from the socket.

Some people are granted advantages in life at birth. Few had come to Danny. He was born with severe hemophilia. As a child, physical abuse at the hands of his father dulled his brain, but not his irrepressible personality. His mother? I met her once and heard her tearful accounts of the children she was fostering at that time. However, although living in Spokane, Washington, she never visited Danny in the time I knew him. Not once. She did not call. He had a younger brother, damaged but less so, who despite his hemophilia, was able to hold jobs, marry, and begin a family. The brothers remained on good terms. Like many disabled adults, Danny did not have a legal guardian. The staff at the Puget Sound Blood Center stepped in and assisted with case management needs.

Danny lived in a series of facilities - his odyssey through them reflected his mix of real limits masked by prominent social skills, genuine friendliness, and some degree of shrewdness and persistence. He made some friends in these facilities. Among them were folks who frequented social service agencies, and the local public hospital. When frustrated, however, by his own limitations, less-than-helpful caregivers, or by his inability to do things by himself, some combativeness and temper would emerge, and we would wonder about a need to begin planning again.

Independent in the use public transportation and his own scooter, Danny would wheel into the Blood Center frequently for infusions, consultations, or just to joke and hang out. He was respectful of our time, and would not interrupt anything that was going on. The hemophilia staff and other Blood Center staff looked forward to his visits, understood him, and made a fuss over him. But if someone he wanted to talk to was unavailable, he would pout, turn up his nose, pretend he didn't care, and then repeatedly ask when that person would be available. It wasn't just the hemophilia staff that loved and cared about him – everyone loved him – the security guards, reception staff, and folks from other parts of the Blood Center who saw him wheeling around. We were a safe haven for him. He would wheel past the staff's doors, peer in if he could, and start a conversation or make a joke. Danny loved his providers outside of the PSBC, too, including his orthopedist and his internal medicine specialist. He would simply glow at their attention and interest. Under the guidance of a student nurse, one year he made everyone a Valentine's Day card and dropped them off at our offices. It was an emotional day as he shyly wheeled around dropping off his cards, relishing the happiness and gratitude of those who so appreciated his effort. Our receptionist burst into tears which only added to his happiness.

Danny's friendliness to us did not extend too far beyond the boundaries of our facility. Outside of the PSBC, he wanted to maximize his independence and have his medical integrity remain confidential. Running into him on the street, he would ignore us as interlopers into his secret world. I think he treasured the moments with people from other worlds, wanting to be considered normal or, at least, less impaired. Outside of the PSBC, we were embarrassing to him.

There were a lot of struggles. Danny was always on the edge of fully comprehending the world, and his jokes and unpredictable responses to those who were not aware of his limits or his defensiveness sometimes caused a public fracas. Keeping him safe definitely took a village. For a time, he lived in an adult care home. Unprepared for the complexity of his care and his bellicose outbursts, the managers of the house limited his access to the residence when they were not present. As a consequence, he was occasionally locked out of the house, leaving him to wait for their return in Seattle's famously wet weather. We helped him find a new place, and I attended a hearing about his previous caregivers and recommended they no longer be allowed to care for HIV+ individuals.

Eligible for a handicapped bus pass, he would occasionally get into verbal scrapes with testy bus drivers or passengers. In between escapades, Danny hung out with friends, including a special friend who was a patient at PSBC. He was always seeking contact and reaching out. He knew about his own disorders and was cooperative with treatment. His health care was good, but his overall health was failing, and he needed greater levels of care.

One of his most engaging features was his delight with any treat, any recognition.

Birthday party–As Danny's 40th birthday approached, we decided to give him a birthday party. We made a big fuss but didn't tell Danny what was going on – simply ordering him not to enter the room that we had set up. Of course, all he wanted to do was enter the room. He was delighted, questioning, and asking us what was going on. The big moment came and Ta-Dum!– we ushered him into the room to see his cake, receive his presents, and sing some songs. He was thrilled, and I still treasure that moment.

Hospice–As his health failed and his care needs escalated, he moved into a local hospice. Relationships there mirrored other contacts he had had. His roughness alienated some people. To others, he was connected.

Trip–For someone who had known so little, he was excited at the prospect of a hospice- sponsored excursion to an overnight camp on Washington's Olympic Peninsula with a group of hospice residents. To some this might have been daunting, but not to Danny. Unequipped with items such as a suitcase, or the means to purchase a bag, he tossed some clothing into a black plastic trash bag. Returning from the trip, he was glowing! He never told us what he experienced there, but he loved it. With the biggest of grins, he said he wanted to move there!

We became aware during one of Danny's hospitalizations of a hospice volunteer named Tom who was a gentle, elderly man, endlessly patient, who loved working with Danny. Tom spent time with him and took him out for excursions. We all marveled at Tom's sociability, his responsiveness, and his willingness to connect. Eventually Danny talked a little about Tom, and we were allowed to meet this compassionate and caring soul. Also at the hospice was a lady with whom Danny bonded and he wanted to marry her. His romantic plan was sadly interrupted by her illness and subsequent death. Although Danny's activities at hospice were mostly secret, we appreciated the things he did share with us.

Tom was with Danny when he died. His funeral was well attended by members of his extended clan, many of whom bore a distinct resemblance to him. People drove from the Midwest, even from across the country, to honor him. His funeral ended with some moments of pure astonishment when a bagpipe player split the air in the small church. Danny's mother, on continuous oxygen, wheezed away while his father appeared stoic. I felt very sad that Danny's parents never got to see, or understand, his special sense of humor or his struggles to belong. His greatest desires were to become a member of a group, to push beyond his limits, to show kindness toward his friends, and to embrace life.

Well, Danny, please know that a lot of us did understand. We miss you still.

Susan Kocik, MSW, LCSW
Seattle, Washington

Paralyzed But Not Broken

He was a little over a year old and had no idea how his life would unfold. He was born into a very poor Hispanic family with non-English speaking parents. Laying on an emergency room table in a government-funded hospital, scared and crying, he received his first infusion of factor concentrate.

For the sake of anonymity, I will refer to him as Rey. I met Rey at my Treatment Center when he was almost 16 years old. He was an average student in the 10th grade. After school and on weekends Rey was learning the trade of remodeling houses. He made some extra money helping his cousins remodel bathrooms and doing handiwork in very nice, expensive homes in and around the city he grew up in. All the while he never had a real place to call home. The stabilizing force in his life was his grandmother. She traveled back and forth between Mexico and the US staying in each country for extended periods of time. His father was around, but not present, so he learned to raise himself. But I am getting ahead of myself so let's go back to the beginning.

You see, that one year old beautiful baby boy was abandoned by his mother. She returned to Mexico where she is currently living. His maternal grandmother took him in and along with a part-time father, Rey grew up in a lower socioeconomic neighborhood near the U.S.-Mexico border in Texas. Rey speaks both English (fluently) and Spanish which is his first language. At sixteen years old I found Rey to be well-mannered, polite, and soft spoken. I would see him only at clinic visits (when he would remember to come) and always when he needed factor. Rey was mostly happy, never once complaining about having been dealt a tough hand in life. There were no homemade cookies waiting for him after school, no safe neighborhood to play in, and very little factor VIII concentrate available to give him to stop his bleeds.

Rey is not a legal U.S. citizen. As you might imagine, treating bleeds was a challenge, factor was scarce, and when we did find some factor to give him, it didn't work. Rey had developed an inhibitor after his first few infusions of factor concentrate sixteen years earlier.

While living part time with some extended family members, going to school, and working on the side, Rey woke up one morning with a bleed in his back caused by a protruding spring from the second-hand sofa he was sleeping on. Having no factor to treat the bleed, he went to a local emergency room for medical care. He walked with great difficulty through the electric sliding emergency room doors, crying in pain. What the hospital staff saw that day was a large, young Hispanic man walking in through their emergency room door with no insurance, no money to pay for his care, and no legal right to be in this country. He waited in pain, sitting on a hard, plastic chair which was fastened to five other chairs, all with someone sitting in them who was either hurting or bleeding. They were all waiting with anticipation to see a medical person who would provide them care.

Several hours later he met with an intern and tried to answer the many questions being asked of him. He explained his situation, asked for help with the pain, and told the intern he had hemophilia. During his conversation with the intern, it became clear to Rey that he was a burden to this intern, that he was an expense to the hospital, and that he was being completely judged for not being born in the city he grew up in and in the only country he knew. After what seemed like hours, Rey was admitted to the hospital and treated for his pain. Dozing off and waking up when someone would enter his hospital room, he tried to talk to whoever would listen. He kept telling them, "I have hemophilia!" The hospital personnel took his blood, they took his blood pressure, they took his temperature, and even took his urine, but they never once took him at his word.

It seemed like the next evening when Rey woke up in a dark room with a new awareness that there was another person in the bed next to him moaning and crying for help. He reached for his call button in an effort to assist, but could not find it anywhere. He wanted to tell his new roommate he would call for help, but the moaning overpowered his words, leaving Rey feeling even more helpless. Rey found the light over his bed and turned it on deciding to walk to the nurse's station to get help. He wasn't feeling any pain now so moving would be easier. Rey pulled back the sheets, opened his mouth and yelled, "I need help!" Rey couldn't feel his legs. After too many hours in the hospital without any treatment for his bleed, Rey was paralyzed from the waist down. Rey had no way of knowing that the last time he would ever walk was the day he entered the hospital emergency room bent over in pain with a bleed in his spine.

I have spent the last 14 years helping Rey find quality in his life. I talked him down off the ledge a few times and visited him in the hospital after two attempts at suicide. I found him treatment where I could, pushed him to get a GED, and tried to give him hope when he had none. I still see Rey at clinic when he comes. I have met his beautiful wife and helped them find furniture for their apartment. I am waiting for the day when he becomes a citizen of the only country he's ever known and loved. I am waiting for the day when Rey can get the needed treatment and care he deserves without barriers. Rey doesn't talk any more about that back bleed so many years ago. He accepts his life as it is and looks for ways to find joy and hope. As for me, I struggle with the ignorance and neglect that Rey endured when his back bleed went untreated. I struggle with the discrimination and prejudice that so often impede good treatment and care. I struggle with knowing this should never have happened to Rey. Sometimes it seems that I am the one paralyzed and in need of hope.

Ed Kuebler, MSW, LCSW
Houston, Texas

The Marksman

In 1998, while working for the Hemophilia Foundation of Illinois, I had the opportunity to work with a contingent of about twenty patients who were accessing services at Michael Reese Hospital in Chicago, Illinois. Michael Reese Hospital was located just south of "The Loop" and most of their pediatric and adult patients were from the City of Chicago.

Most of my patients were co-infected with HIV and Hepatitis C. Some had lost brothers and relatives. Their outlook on life was not good. I tried to encourage these young men to think short-term and not long-term. My clinical skills were very limited because I had attended social work graduate school in the administration track. There were medications in the research pipeline. I encouraged my patients not to give up; to keep the faith.

I also encountered a young man named Marcus. He was a teenager with severe hemophilia A and co-infected. His outlook on life was slightly different from some of my older patients. Marcus had become a counselor, then a senior counselor at the annual hemophilia summer camp, which lasted a week. A few parents and I began transporting many of the inner- city boys to camp and picking them up a week later. Marcus and I would have some deep discussions about life during and after some of these excursions. Of course, I would have my Motown cruising music. Marcus and his friends asked if I would play some of their music, which I reluctantly agreed to do. When we had dropped everyone off at their destinations, Marcus asked me the most profound question that I had heard: "Do you listen to the words and to what the person is trying to say?" I learned to listen.

Marcus shared with me that he had begun to DJ on the weekends. He told me his Dad required him to be available for church every Sunday morning. No problem. Marcus had learned to play the keyboards by watching and listening to others; a gift. He had also begun to record some of his music and lyrics. I encouraged him to write and record about his medical issues, which he did wholeheartedly. He also wrote lyrics to express his frustration with fellow counselors who he had befriended and who took jobs as homecare representatives.

I can't prove it, or have any data on this, but Marcus and two of his friends stopped going to camp after the summer of 2004. They passed away in the following successive years: 2005, 2006, and 2007. Why? They stopped taking their medications. Had they entered into a pact? I don't know.

Marcus was a very resilient young man who blessed us with HIV and Hepatitis C prevention songs that are used nationwide. He was fondly referred to as "The Marksman". I loved the Marksman: my patient, my youngest son.

Greg McClure, BA, MA, MS, LSW
Chicago, Illinois

I Remember ...

When I think of the legacy left to the hemophilia community because of the HIV/AIDS epidemic, I think of those patients who most profoundly inspired me during those years. I think of Jim, Cara, Joseph, Vicki, Matthew, Nathan, Sally, Fred, John, Bill, Allan, Ben and Noah not to mention the twins, Randy and Andy among many others. I am left reflecting on how they touched me, and what they taught me throughout those years. Taught me? Hmm. I smile and say, "thank you." Why? Because ...

Through those years of being involved in the lives of these patients, I was allowed a peek into the mystery of living, dying, leaving legacies, and eternity. They showed so much courage and ferocity in their efforts to overcome AIDS and to live. I was in awe and now acknowledge that they have given me a wisdom and strength I would not otherwise have. They showed me how much control we humans have over the moment we transition into another realm and how when the time came, how very unique and individualistic the death experience was for each of them. They fought to live and they fought hard, but eventually they just realized they were very tired of fighting. Not long after reaching that point, I saw how they "decided" to just "let go." For some, it was so obvious that they literally exercised choice in the matter. I mean, who would have thought?

Having given birth to two children and being present for the births of my grandchildren, I appreciated these patients allowing me a glimpse of a phenomenon I now refer to as "reverse birth." Let me explain. There is a PROCESS in birthing, and there is a PROCESS in dying. With birth, you are not here, and then you are. With death, you are here, and then you are not. Just like that! During the birth process, the mother and the baby must endure labor and the experience of pain and suffering before the baby is born. And then, for just a moment, as the baby's head emerges...a pause. A quiet moment. During the process of death, the person labors long and experiences pain and suffering. He or she may cry out (and certainly those around them do)...just before they die. Just at the moment when the heart ceases beating, there's a pause, a second of peace, and then quiet. But, unlike what many think about dying, that moment is neither painful, nor terrible. Some patients, with whom I spent their final moments, described their joy at the beauty of what they were seeing. They saw Jesus, an angel, or an already deceased relative coming for them. Some felt there really was a place to which they were going, and they relaxed and even smiled. I am very grateful and have found much comfort in these insight-producing moments.

As I reflect now, I feel humbled I had the privilege of being a part of my patients' journeys. They experienced intense anger about the hand they had been unjustly dealt. They moved through their anger to a sense of resignation. Finally they found the courage, in the last months of their lives, to accept death head on. At that point, so many of those named above demonstrated the strength and the will to live the rest of their young lives with courage, wisdom, and insight. They had a depth of spirit that one would think is generally reserved for the elderly. As I talked with them and their families over the months of their illnesses, I often wondered how on earth, if I were faced with the same set of circumstances, would I be able to handle what they were forced to endure? I still don't know the answer because I've never been gravely ill or experienced death. But I do know this. I know I CAN do it if I have to, because they did it! My patients have been my teachers and our relationships will live in my heart for the rest of my life. I will never, ever forget them or what they have given me. I now know that dying is not all that bad. It is just a part of life, and in the end, it will come to us all. So I'd best accept that and get on with living life to the fullest!

Finally, I wish I could tell my patients there were many

reasons for their lives on this earth. What they brought to their families and to those who loved them was irreplaceable. Beyond that, their tragedy raised an unexpected awareness of this obscure population. The voices of those with bleeding disorders would have otherwise just whistled in the wind. In turn, this awareness translated into the unprecedented efficacy and purity of products for treating bleeding disorders. And there is more to come. Their sacrifice made hemophilia care and treatment what it is today. Patients now enjoy the benefits of amazing education, care, and treatment. In the mid-1980's, in response to HIV/AIDS, federally funded hemophilia treatment centers raised care and treatment to a much higher level. Patients are now almost totally free of joint disease and other historical complications. How different treatment and care would be today, were it not for the United States becoming aware of people with hemophilia as a result of HIV/AIDS. This is their legacy which we must never forget!

Danna Merritt, MSW, LMSW
Detroit, Michigan

Carter's Journey

Today was the yearly Zoo Event, organized by the Calgary Hemophilia Chapter for families with children with hemophilia. It was a grey rainy day and we were running around trying to find some shelter from the rain while directing families to the big white tent where exciting activities were about to take place.

As I was searching for parents and children at the entrance to the zoo, I noticed that a little person was holding my hand. I looked down and saw a beautiful face with a big smile and two big eyes looking up at me with anticipation. Carter, a four year old boy who was diagnosed with severe FVIII deficiency, was patiently waiting to be taken for an adventure tour of the Siberian tigers as we were running between the raindrops. I was about to discover Carter.

Carter is a vibrant, active four year old boy that I met during the family's first visit at the Hemophilia Clinic when he was one month old. Willie and his wife, Jennifer, were referred to the clinic after prolonged bleeding following Carter's circumcision. Jennifer had a five year old daughter earlier and everything went fairly smooth during her birth. For this reason, she did not suspect anything when giving birth to Carter. She was released from the hospital the next day and was sent home.

On the fourth week Carter had an appointment for a circumcision and Jennifer took him to the hospital by herself. She was told that circumcision was a simple procedure and for this reason she decided to handle it by herself. Following the procedure, Jennifer decided to spend some quality time with her daughter Cassie. With the onset of Carter's birth, Jennifer felt depressed and sad. Cassie, who until this time did not have to share her mother with a noisy little baby, felt lonely and neglected. The day, however, did not go smoothly. Carter was bleeding following circumcision and the family rushed the child to the hospital thinking, "The doctor ruined our son." A few hours after being at the hospital and thinking the worst, Jennifer was told the test results showed that Carter had moderate hemophilia.

The family came to the hemophilia clinic a week later. My first impression was that although the couple seemed anxious and overwhelmed with their baby's new diagnosis, they tried to hide their feelings and look calm. Looking back, I can only imagine how profoundly difficult it was for the parents to hear their baby had a rare bleeding disorder which they had never heard about before. It reminded me of my reaction when I started working in hemophilia. The first thing I thought was, "What is hemophilia?" I had never heard about this disease before. Little did I know the impact that this condition would have on the everyday life of a parent, a child, and the family.

During the meeting the couple was told, among other things, the lab had made a mistake and Carter had severe Type A hemophilia and not moderate hemophilia. As I was observing the parents' reaction, it was clear they did not trust the team. I was not surprised when they asked for a second test to make sure their child had an accurate diagnosis. Deep inside they were hoping he did not have hemophilia.

During the long meeting, the team handed the family a binder filled with information and each team member provided them with some education and answered a few questions. We all knew, however, that it would take many months before Jennifer and Willie could cope with Carter's medical condition. In the next few months, Jennifer often visited our clinic to obtain more information and to discuss issues she emotionally could not handle. She had difficulty coping with Carter's new diagnosis and spent months in a state of depression. She was angry that she was not able to protect her child from bleeding and felt anxious about her own test result showing that she was a carrier.

Joining the family in this process, I was constantly learning, as a hemophilia social worker, about the impact of the diagnosis on their daily lives. Through their experience, this family was teaching me how the love for your child can change the way you view life and function in this world. The process can be long and painful.

Jennifer was in complete denial for a long period of time until one day Carter had his first bleed. He rolled over on a toy and bruised his back near his kidney area. This was a moment of awakening for Jennifer. At that moment, she knew she needed to help her son and to admit for the first time that her child had hemophilia. From being passive and depressed, Jennifer was able to transform herself and become an active participant in advocating for her son and other people with bleeding disorders. She immersed herself with information, attended the Hemophilia Society events, met other parents during conferences and workshops, and talked to anyone who was willing to listen about what she knew about the disorder.

Jennifer armed her son with a helmet and knee pads and went through the painful experience of learning how to infuse Carter at home without the use of a port. She was very proud of herself. Jennifer did not stop there, however. She joined the Southern Alberta Chapter of the Hemophilia Society Board and attended, with her husband Willie, the Parents Empowering Parents (PEP) workshop facilitated by the hemophilia team. She became one of the parent leaders. She created a website and events to raise money for the Hemophilia Society and was the co-founder of "Carter's Quest."

I was in awe! How is it that parents can move from such a time of devastation to a time of strength, motivation, and advocacy? Where did she draw this energy from? I have been working with Jennifer since Carter's birth, and while many would have thought, "She is going crazy," I sensed a strong determination from a mother with an abundance of love for her child. Through this experience, I am constantly reminded of the strength of a parent's love for their child and the need to support the parents to make positive changes and outcomes.

Four years later, Jennifer accepts Carter's medical condition. She also understands that she cannot change the journey her family had to take when Carter was born. She cannot take away the pain that Carter and his family may experience throughout their lives. Nevertheless, Jennifer is a proud mother and a great example for other parents who have had similar experiences.

When you approach Jennifer she always smiles and says, "We are not special people but we love our kids, and Carter is no exception. Aside from his underlying condition, he is a normal little kid who loves to cuddle, loves to jump, and gets hurt."

Discovering Carter enabled me to discover the social worker within myself. The journey with Carter continues to remind me daily of the importance of believing in families and their ability to move beyond the difficulties to make a difference for their loved ones. To Jennifer, Carter, and their family...I am grateful.

Hulda Niv, MSW, RSW
Calgary, Alberta, Canada

Santiago

Santiago was one of the first patients I met. I was new to hemophilia and it was my first month in the position.

I hadn't had much luck with outreach to the community. The HTC had been without a social worker for a year and a half and the patients had gotten on with their lives. One day, Santiago happened to come to the hospital for tests and he agreed to sit down to talk with me. He was a man in his early 40's, attractive, well dressed, and soft spoken. Anyone looking at him would think that there wasn't anything particularly wrong with him. He was a very private person and was reluctant to talk at first. But somehow we both felt a connection and after a while he told me his story.

Santiago was the youngest of 10 children, five boys and five girls. He was the only one with hemophilia. He was born into a working class Mexican/American family. His father came from Mexico as a young man and his mother was from a U.S. border town. His father worked in construction and sometimes worked three different jobs a day to support his family and pay for Santiago's medical care. His mother, a stay-at-home mom, ruled the household with a velvet fist, cooking, cleaning, and caring for the children. They lived in a modest home on the south side of Tucson. It was a happy family that dealt with life's challenges with laughter and love.

The late 1960's were the years before prophylaxis. The treatment was cryoprecipitate and for Santiago, this meant going to the hospital three times a week. He told me that his father would come home after working a 12 hour day, eat dinner and take him to the hospital. Frequently, this would mean a 4-5 hour hospital stay and they wouldn't get home until after midnight. Perhaps because of this, Santiago developed a unique relationship with his dad. It was his dad that he remembers sitting at his bedside, his dad who helped protect him from harm. And it was his dad, who in an attempt to give him "normal" experiences, took him walking in the woods and taught him to shoot a gun and hunt. This is not to say that his mother wasn't a large part of his life. She was his nurturer at home. She volunteered at his school and chauffeured the kids. But it was with his father that he felt a special bond.

Santiago's generation was hit hard by the HIV/AIDS epidemic. If you were lucky to survive those years, you seldom came through them unscathed. He told me how when he was small, the doctors told his parents that due to his hemophilia, he probably wouldn't live to be ten years old. When he survived into his late teens and got HIV from the contaminated blood supply, the doctors told him that his life expectancy, due to his HIV, would be short. When he survived living with HIV, got older, and hemophilia treatment improved, the doctors told him that the worst was now over and he should go out and live. As Santiago told his story, I couldn't help but wonder how foreign all that must have seemed. He was one of a generation of men with hemophilia who were told for most of their lives that they were going to die. Now they were being told to go out and live? How were they supposed to do that?

As Santiago grew and reached adulthood, he finished high school, became an EMT and an LPN. He got a job working in direct patient care in a renal dialysis center. He loved his job, felt he was finally giving back, but then lost his job when the administration found out he had HIV. It was the end of the 1980's. Fear was high and understanding was poor. It was, in short, the dark ages.

When I first met Santiago, he was going through a divorce and was seeking joint custody of his 3 children. He was living with his elderly parents and was proud to be their main caregiver. His health was declining due to co-morbidities of HIV, Hepatitis C, and renal insufficiency. Although he looked healthy, he was frequently tired and the battle for his children was demanding much of his strength and finances. He continued to slowly decline. His kidneys weren't working. Dialysis was offered but he declined and went on hospice. The roles switched again and his parents became his caregiver. During this time I made weekly visits. Frequently, when entering his room, I would see his elderly father sitting at his bedside. I couldn't help but think about how many times this man had done this. How familiar this all must feel. Here was the son he would always protect from harm, in a larger body, perhaps, but still his little boy.

When Santiago was sleeping or too weak to talk, I'd sit with his parents. They'd tell me family stories and tales of his childhood. Santiago's relatives, brothers and sisters, aunts and uncles, nieces and nephews who'd come to visit would also share their stories. We'd sit at the kitchen table and laugh and cry together. I came to relish my visits and was in awe of his loving, supportive family. I was amazed at how they had coped with all this tragedy and how they kept strong and united.

After a year and a half, something strange started to happen. Santiago started to get better. His kidney function was still poor, but his mentation cleared. He woke up one day and wanted to start driving. We were all apoplectic! He continued to improve. He started with physical therapy. He began to walk and lo and behold, he started to drive!

At this writing, Santiago is very much alive. He has renewed a relationship with his eldest daughter and she is now living with him and going to college. She wants to become a nurse. He is driving and has returned to be the main caregiver for his aging parents. I visited him several days ago to get his permission to write this story. While I was sitting there I silently reflected on how many lifetimes this man has had. How many predictions of death he has survived. He is a child of hemophilia's "lost generation"; the generation of old treatment methods, contaminated blood supplies, HIV, AIDS, and Hepatitis A, B and C. But Santiago is a survivor and he has definitely survived.

ADDENDUM: MAY, 2013

As social workers, we know the one sure thing in life is change.

Several weeks after I wrote this story, Santiago started to decline. First, his stamina decreased, then his body retained extra fluid, and finally he became jaundiced. Treatment was useless, unable to cure the evils that had bombarded his system for 47 years. It was time to talk hospice. Santiago knew it. In a conversation we had prior to his admittance into hospice he said, "I remember my previous time in hospice. I just know that this time the end result won't be the same." He was right. Santiago died at home in the same room he had grown up in.

Sometimes, no matter how long we live or how far we travel, we end up coming back to where we started.

Laurel Pennick, MSSW, LCSW
Tucson, Arizona

Brief Encounter—Lifetime Impact

I don't remember his name. My contact with him was very brief. But his impact on me lasted forever. I had just accepted a position at University of Missouri Hospital. My duties included pediatric oncology, sickle cell, cleft palate, and neurosurgery, plus both pediatric and adult hematology. Even with twenty-five years of experience as a social worker, there was a lot to learn in my new position. Learning came quickly during the first adult hematology clinic when I met a man with a bleeding disorder who had a profound effect on my values.

He regrettably grew up when bleeding disorders were treated with human blood products. During one of these treatments he contracted HIV. This became a huge issue when administrators at the school where he taught fired him. They shared the prevailing prejudice at the time that this virus could spread easily and infect others. I asked the patient how he handled such a devastating stigma caused by prejudices that were prevalent among much of society at that time. Even though he innocently contracted this virus and did not deserve such discrimination, he did not exhibit any resentment. I, however, being in the profession of Social Work where we are taught to fight injustice, was angry. How could such a caring and innocent man be subjected to such bias? My response was vindictive. I strongly suggested that he sue the school district for unlawful termination. His response was more forgiving. He did not want to want to take any legal action and did not blame the administrators because they were influenced by society's bigotry. His response that day taught me more about tolerance and acceptance than all the books and classes from my years of education.

My next contact with this patient came almost a year later. He was in the intensive care unit at University of Missouri Hospital. The virus was devastating his body and he was close to dying. Even then, he did not blame anyone or hold resentments. He died during that hospitalization. My contact with him was brief, but his impact on my life was unending. He taught me a lot about acceptance, trust, and caring. His lessons influenced my contacts with other patients throughout my social work career and have had a significant impact on my personal values.

Wayne Richards, MSW, LCSW
Columbia, Missouri

Reflections of a Retired HTC Social Worker

For nearly twenty years, until my 2003 retirement, I was the Hemophilia Treatment Center (HTC) social worker at Children's Hospital Oakland (CHO). It's hard to believe this year is the 10th anniversary of my retirement. The invitation to contribute to this collection is an opportunity to reflect on those two decades of medical advances in hemophilia care, progress in patient autonomy, and the impact of HIV/AIDS on the bleeding disorders community.

In my early forties and fresh out of graduate school following an MSW internship at CHO, I was hired to be the CHO/HTC social worker. I knew almost nothing about hemophilia, but what I *thought* I knew was patently wrong. As luck would have it, I joined a group of experienced and collaborative practitioners. They recommended reading material, referred me to knowledgeable social workers in the HTC network, *and* to patients and their parents who were included as contributors on the multidisciplinary HTC team. These resources brought me up to speed. Over the years, even as the cast of HTC players changed, I was frequently reminded of my good fortune to learn from, and work with, a team of extraordinary professionals along with patients and their families.

Graduate school courses and my internships prepared me for the social work role and team colleagues educated me about CHO systems, hemophilia, von Willebrand's Disease, and other bleeding disorders. As the team social worker, the experts I most relied on were the patients and families, the people with first-hand experience living with a bleeding disorder. From day one, I learned about the extraordinary spirit and understanding of even very young children, like the 5 year-old "unaffected" sister of a toddler with severe hemophilia. She explained, "whenever our family plans an outing or vacation, we always have a contingency plan just in case my little brother has a bleed." Her disclosure let me know her whole family was "affected", not just her brother who had hemophilia. The family's candid communication and anticipatory planning normalized hemophilia and reduced the potential for resentment when unavoidable bleeding episodes disrupted their plans.

Often, families with a history of severe hemophilia lacked information about the treatment advances since their affected relative's childhood. Understandably, parents feared their son might face the same physical pain, damaged joints, activity limits, lifetime dependency, and discrimination that a maternal grandfather, cousin, or uncle might have confronted. Justifiably, many young parents were anxious about insurance coverage, periodic school absences, exclusion from peer activities, future employability, and more. Regardless of their child's HIV status, they feared AIDS, the public's association of the disease with hemophilia, and general ignorance about HIV transmission risks. Similarly, families totally blindsided by the diagnosis feared a dreadfully restricted future for their son, the impact on siblings who did not have hemophilia, and the possibility their daughters were carriers.

Despite divergent cultural backgrounds, experiences, and histories, families who met at clinic visits and at Hemophilia Foundation of Northern California (HFNC) events, developed relationships reminiscent of reunions among long-lost relatives. I witnessed the benefits of these interdependent relationships and learned to appreciate, and actively promote, peer support. Indeed, common concerns and a desire for a sense of community inspired me to conceive of a weekend family camp. For several years, families collaborated on all aspects of the program. During the year prior to my retirement, leadership of the camp transitioned to empowered community members and the HFNC. The very popular annual Family Camp thrives as a place where multigenerational families socialize, participate in education sessions, and learn from peers.

The life-threatening health consequences of HIV/AIDS and Hepatitis C infections are well documented. So, too, is the fear of infection from clotting factor, fear of disclosure, fear of transmission, fear of discrimination, exclusion, and denial of access to school. This collective anxiety dominated the community for years. News coverage of Ryan White's mistreatment justified these fears. Parents of youngsters seen at CHO's pediatric HTC were overwhelmed by information and weighed down by the absence of treatment for their infected children. For those electing to have a child tested, the uncertainty of whether to inform the child was a difficult decision.

One of CHO's memorable patients took the matter into his own bold hands. When Jack (not his real name), a regular at summer camp and a popular role model, was in the 5th, or perhaps 6th grade, he wrote in his class journal about his HIV+ status. Subsequently, his school's principal, a district nurse, Jack's teacher, his parents, Dana Francis (the social worker at the Hemophilia Council of California), and I attended a "planning meeting" to consider how to proceed. Prior to Jack's disclosure, the school district had no policies regarding HIV+ students.

What I most remember was Jack's extraordinary confidence and his control of the meeting. Collaborative decisions were made about how to protect and ensure his privacy and optimize safety for other children. I believe Jack matured as an empowered public spokesman on behalf of persons with HIV/AIDS *because* he had hemophilia – not *despite* having hemophilia. When he was a young teen and terminally ill with HIV-related illnesses, Jack made the decision to receive only comfort care. His courage, in the face of adversity, was inspirational. He influenced peers who had been less active in the bleeding disorders community to become involved advocates and mentors for other youngsters.

My twenty years as the CHO/HTC social worker spanned a time of great treatment advances, one of the worst medical catastrophes imaginable, *and* extraordinary advocacy by the affected community. The development of factor concentrates, interventions for the treatment of disabling inhibitors, and increased appreciation for patients' rights and responsibilities, improved care immeasurably. The concentrates made it possible for people with hemophilia to live independently, travel, and maintain normal daily routines. Immune tolerance regimens radically changed lives. Just one example is the then 11 year-old CHO patient who presented with a debilitating inhibitor to FVIII that was successfully overridden by immune tolerance therapy. He's now a 22 year-old University of California graduate. In the fall of this year, he will be a first-year student at a prestigious medical school.

One of the most high profile accomplishments during my tenure was the community's response to the egregious behavior of the factor manufacturers. The determination of a committed group of advocates and their allies ultimately uncovered truths and corporate liability for HIV infection in people with bleeding disorders. The HIV/AIDS experience, disastrous as it certainly was, and is for the infected individuals who still thrive, empowered patients to be proactive on behalf of their healthcare.

While no longer immersed in the world of bleeding disorders, I still have powerful memories of the extraordinary courage and resilience of the families I had the privilege to know over the course of 20 years. Their capacity to live successfully with a chronic health condition was often awe-inspiring. I remain indebted to the families who taught me many important life lessons.

Bobbie Steinhart, MSW
Berkeley, California

The Spirit of Endurance

I have come to learn that the spirit of endurance is exemplified in individuals living with a chronic condition. I would like to share experiences I have encountered in working in the hemophilia community. The first one takes place here in the United States, in our Hemophilia Treatment Center, (HTC). The other experience was with a group of individuals I met in South America. These stories have shown me that resilience, determination, and endurance have no limits, especially for those living with a chronic medical condition like hemophilia. When these individuals make up their minds, there is little that they can't achieve.

Roger came to see us at the HTC in a wheelchair. In spite of his limitations, he was happy and very polite. His smile could light up the room! When the team met this young man, everyone kept saying what a remarkable and well-adjusted person he was. In spite of all his medical challenges and limitations, Roger was "standing tall" in his wheelchair. Roger shared with us that he had completed college in his native country and was looking forward to entering the work force as an architect. He had adapted to being in the wheelchair and shared that he thought he would always be in a wheelchair.

Growing up, Roger had limited factor to treat his bleeds. His family attended to his needs and provided support by applying cold compresses, keeping him off his feet, and limiting his mobility in an attempt to lessen his pain and injuries. Roger and his family were doing all they could, but the damage going on inside his joints was beginning to limit his movement. After a period of time he ended up in the wheelchair with severe atrophy of both his legs.

The very first time we saw Roger he was evaluated by our entire team; doctor, nurse, physical therapist, and social worker.

After the examination, the family was told that with regular factor infusions and physical therapy, there was a strong possibility this young man would be able to walk again. The wheelchair could be used when needed along with other devices that would provide assistance for him to walk. Roger's eyes welled with tears and both he and his mother were crying with joy because there was hope! The idea of walking again was so important to him.

Roger had a positive outcome following our team's recommendations. With a strict regimen of physical therapy and exercise (which he followed religiously), and his medications, Roger was able to walk, at first with a walker, and then with crutches. He still uses the wheelchair when he has a "bad bleed." He has a positive attitude about walking again. Treatment, and just "plain old endurance", in spite of a difficult chronic illness, has changed his life for the better.

In South America I met a group of men of different ages. Some were in their teens, twenties, thirties, and fifties. The man in his fifties created a remarkable impression when he said he was employed full time even though you could clearly see the damage in all of his joints and the difficulties with his movements. He shared he had been very lucky not to have gotten factor in his younger years because of the crisis of HIV. There was also a young man who shared that he could not hold a regular job because of his medical condition since sometimes he was not able to ambulate. This young man had started his own small business. On the days when he felt well, he sold pre-paid cell phones and cards at the local bus depot. He, too, had a wonderful smile. To this day I still remember him. He gave me the strong impression that he was grateful about life in general.

While in Peru, on the day we had clinic, there was a young child whose mother was carrying him on her back. You could clearly see that this child was about six or seven years old but he was still being carried by his mother. Later on when we met this handsome child, we learned this woman and her child had traveled nine hours by bus to meet the medical team who treated his hemophilia. The mother carried the child because of the damage he had endured due to bleeds, no factor, and the very limited medical care available to the family. We also found out the family lived in the remote highlands of Peru. The child's father worked in the mines and came to see his family twice a month. The family lived in a lower part of the mountains where the mother attended to the family and their livestock on a small plot of land. Things were looking up for the family as they would soon have medical insurance through the father's employer. The family would have access to medications and treatment, but the long traveling distance would still be a problem.

I need to mention that when the physical therapist was examining the child and explaining to the mother how to apply ice to a bleed, the mother's facial expression was as if to say "how do I get the ice?" Yes, there was ice nearby where they lived, but it was not readily available. The physical therapist quickly understood there was no refrigerator in the home and explained to the mother that she could use cold water compresses to help her son.

As I write these memories of meeting all these wonderful individuals, I remember the imprints they left on my heart. Seeing their determination to hold jobs, to continue their education, and to just simply "live their lives" has made me think about their "spirit of endurance."

Silvia Vega, BA
Los Angeles, California

Jay

I met Jay in March 1995, two months after I started in my position as the Hemophilia Social Worker at the UConn Hemostasis and Thrombosis Center. He was 36 years old and a member of the generation of individuals with hemophilia who had been infected with HIV from blood products prior to 1982. During our first encounter, he impressed me as a hard-working and positive person. In spite of his multiple diagnoses and chronic pain, he worked full-time, had what he perceived to be strong support from family and friends, and engaged in a hobby he loved, photographing motorcycle races.

In addition to coping with his complicated health issues and his already busy life, Jay had actively researched information about the Ricky Ray Act and the class action lawsuits related to the transmission of HIV in the blood supply. He called to share what he had learned, and encouraged me to pass the information on to others. He was generous in that way.

In the fall of 1998, Jay began to experience numbness and weakness in his legs. By December, he had no use of his legs and little use of his arms or hands. He was admitted to the hospital, where he stayed for two months. He was diagnosed with chronic inflammatory demyelinating polyneuropathy, and the paralysis continued to worsen. It was not known when, or if, Jay would recover.

During that hospitalization, I met with Jay frequently. His courage and fortitude inspired me and all those providing his care. In spite of increasing physical weakness, Jay exhibited equal determination to recover. As I struggled to raise painful issues related to planning for the possibility that he would not regain physical functioning, he talked about rehabilitation. Eventually he began to regain some feeling, then some ability to twitch a finger, then another finger. After two months, he was discharged to a skilled nursing facility, where he would stay until he was strong enough for more intensive rehabilitation.

Throughout the next year, I met with Jay regularly during his follow-up appointments. At each meeting, Jay talked about his progress. Although he was sometimes frustrated by the slow pace of improvement, he was mostly proud and excited about the slightest increase in functioning. He was always hopeful he would make a complete recovery.

By the fall of 1999, one year after his symptoms began, he was walking with the use of braces and had begun to drive. He was looking forward to returning to work. He talked about his disbelief that he was doing so well. Sixteen months after his symptoms began, in spite of the ongoing need for braces to help with walking, and some difficulty using his hands, he was back to work full-time. He was looking forward to engaging in the summer activities he enjoyed.

I still see Jay whenever he comes to the Hemophilia Treatment Center (HTC), for his comprehensive visits. He retired from his full-time job 2004, when his fatigue and pain made it too difficult to continue working. This month, Jay showed me his photos in a recent issue of a motorcycle racing magazine. Although he is frequently unable to negotiate the rugged terrain where the races take place, he goes to the races to take photographs when he feels up to it.

Every time I see Jay, I feel inspired by his strength, determination, and optimism. He is a humble person, and I'm certain he has no idea of his impact on me and others. It is a personal and professional privilege to know him and to work with him. That's why I'm delighted for the opportunity to write this tribute, to share it with him, and to share his inspiring story with others.

Dawn von Mayrhauser, MSW, LCSW
Farmington, Connecticut

About the Contributors

Marilyn August, MSW, LCSW, has been a social worker for 36 years. She worked as the hemophilia social worker in Arizona for 22 years, where she was also the co-director of Camp HONOR, a camp for children with bleeding disorders and their siblings. Since moving to California nine years ago, she has volunteered with chapters in Northern California and attends Camp Hemotion, where she has been a program director as well as a counselor. She continues to work in the hemophilia community as a Community Relations Manager for a biotech company and lives in Concord, California with her husband Rick. She is also proud of her two grown sons in Arizona, as well as a grandson, who is her pride and joy! She loves the outdoors, traveling, hiking, and camping.

Emily E. Czapek, M.D., has been caring for persons with hemophilia for 40+ years. Her main focus has been implementing a true comprehensive care model (CC) that fits with the patient population being served. She earned her Medical Degree from John Hopkins University School of Medicine, did her Residency at Yale New Haven Hospital and Children's Hospital Boston, and her Fellowship at Beth Israel Deaconess Medical Center. She chaired NHF's Standards' Committee that drafted the second of their CC documents. She established the first CC clinics at Children's Memorial Hospital and Cook County Hospital respectively, both in Chicago. In 1988, she moved to Peoria, IL, to expand the Regional CC clinic begun by Dr. Andrew Weiss. While at the center in Peoria, Dr. Czapek addressed two major problems resulting from the scientific advances brought about by factor concentrates. The first was infection with HIV and/ or Hepatitis C. Secondly, a large rise in factor pricing made it unaffordable for "insurance poor" families. In 1999, Dr. Czapek accepted the part-time position of Associate Medical Director of the Rush HTC (Chicago) with focus on establishing a 340B drug program and designing a women's CC clinic. Of her many interests besides hemophilia, her passion is for dogs, especially the Border collie. Yes, she's the one who buys sheep for her dogs! Now one of her border collies multitasks as her mobility service dog. Effective July 1, 2013, she is retiring completely. She is looking forward to spending more time with her dogs and enjoying music, gardening, and various other interests.

Damia Dillard, MSW, LCSW, has enjoyed a career in social work since graduating from CSU-Sacramento in 1999. She is currently employed at UC Davis Medical Center in Sacramento, CA. She is married and the mother of three beautiful daughters who remain her pride and joy. When she is not working, she enjoys church, cooking, baking, taking family trips, and watching her daughters play basketball.

Sue duTreil, PhD, LCSW, is a social worker and an Assistant Professor of Clinical Medicine at the Louisiana Center for Bleeding and Clotting Disorders located at Tulane University Medical School in New Orleans, LA. She earned her MSW and PhD at Tulane University School of Social Work where she majored in Mental Health Direct Services. She has practiced social work for 37 years, and the past 16 have been in hemophilia care. In 1999 she was the first recipient of the National Hemophilia Foundation's Social Work Excellence Fellowship. She has also served as a Parents Empowering Parents Steering Committee Member from 2005 to 2012 and has served as a consultant to that Committee since 2012.

She has conducted research studies on depression in adolescents with hemophilia who were treated with interferon for Hepatitis C, depression in women with bleeding disorders, and adherence to medical treatment in the hemophilia community. She also completed an efficacy study of the Parents Empowering Parents Program. In 2010, Dr. duTreil was named Social Worker of the Year by the National Hemophilia Foundation. She lives in

Metairie, LA , loves to tend her garden, care for her 13 year old cat, File, and spend time on her front porch where neighbors, friends, and relatives stop by to visit.

Donna Fleming, MSSW, began her social work career over 30 years ago. In 1986, she was hired as the social worker and program coordinator for the Kentucky Hemophilia Treatment Centers and left only by force in 2002 when her husband took a job in Indiana. Donna, her husband, Don, and their 16 year old daughter, Annie, currently reside in Beverly, WV.

Dana Francis, MSW, has been a social worker for 30 years. He currently works with people with bleeding disorders at UCSF Medical Center in San Francisco. He has led groups and retreats for adults and teens for many years in an effort to help men and boys develop emotional support and avoid isolation. He lives in nearby Alameda, CA, is happily married to his wife Natalie, and is the proud father of two wonderful sons. He enjoys cycling, traveling, photography, guitar playing, and anything having to do with Bruce Springsteen.

Elizabeth H. Fung, PhD, LCSW, was a senior social worker for 34 years at Children's Memorial Hospital Hemophilia and Bleeding Disorders services until 2012. In June, 2012, the hospital had a name change, at the donor's request. It's now named Lurie Children's Hospital. She currently serves on the Cultural Diversity Working Group of the National Hemophilia Foundation. She is now in private practice, focusing on stress management, at Lincoln Park Psychology Associates in Chicago. She resides in Chicago, IL, loves swimming, goes to concerts, operas, and theater, and participates in the intercessory ministry at her church. She admits to being a workshop junkie and highly recommends spoiling the grandchildren.

Linda Gammage, MSW, LCSW, has been a medical social worker for 30+ years, 16 at the Hemophilia Treatment Center in Peoria, IL. Now "retired", she remains active in the bleeding disorders community serving as founder of the Advanced Clinical Conferences for Social Workers in Bleeding Disorders and chair of the Planning Committee. She is also founder of NHF's Insurance/Reimbursement Social Worker Conferences and is a consultant/chair of the Planning Committee for these conferences. She and husband, Bill, have a son and two grandsons. She enjoys bird watching, reading, and traveling to "out of the way" places.

Peg Geary, MA, MBA, MPH, LCSW, CCM, has been a medical social worker, researcher, and administrator in hospitals for the last 30 years. In her spare time, she loves traveling, reading and spending time with her family and friends. Peg resides in Massachusetts with her husband, Martin, and her two sons, Matthew and Daniel, who are in college.

Chartara Y. Gilchrist, BA, currently resides in Augusta, GA, where she was born and raised, the eldest of six siblings. For almost fourteen years, she has been the adult hemophilia social worker at Georgia Regents University (formerly the Medical College of Georgia) in Augusta, GA. She enjoys travel, gardening, hiking, and holistic nutrition.

Isabel Lin Guzman, MSW, JD, (known as Isabel Lin when she was a hemophilia social worker) is married with three stepchildren and one daughter. After serving as a hemophilia social worker for almost eight years, Isabel went to law school. The wonderful people in the hemophilia community taught her that "life shrinks or expands in proportion to one's courage" (Anais Nin). This was the reason she went to law school. Now living in Chapel Hill with her family, she is an immigration lawyer.

Margaret Halona, MSW, LMSW, retired as the HTC social worker after 19 years with the Ted R. Montoya Hemophilia Program in Albuquerque NM. She currently works for Coram Specialty Infusion as their social worker. Margaret has two adult daughters, three grandchildren, and two grand-dogs. She loves hanging out with her family and friends. Activities that she enjoys are: salsa dancing, traveling, reading, listening to a variety of music, interior decorating, going to her grandchildren's soccer games, and attending artistic/theatrical events.

Mavis Harrop, MSSW, LCSW, has been a social worker for over 40 years in areas of medical and psychiatric social work. She has been at the Vanderbilt HTC in Nashville, TN, since October 1989. She was a member of NHF's Social Work Working Group for four years representing Region IV. She received the NHF Social Worker of the Year Award in 2003. She is an original member of the Advanced Social Work Conference Planning Committee and member of the Parents Empowering Parents (PEP) Steering Committee. She is a former committee member for NHF's Insurance and Reimbursement conferences. She is also a member of NASW. She loves spending time with her dog, Jake, and has an interest in photography, canoeing, walking the beach, and reading. She is an active member of the Anglican/Episcopal church.

Robert E. Johnson, MDiv, MSW, LCSW, has been the hemophilia social worker at Stroger Hospital since July of 1992. He lives with his wife, Ruth, in Forest Park, IL. He is also President of the Friends of Interfaith Encounter Association, a non-profit organization that supports grassroots peacemaking in the Middle East.

Ellen Kachalsky, MSW, LMSW, ACSW, has been the social worker for the Adult Hemophilia Treatment Center for the last 16 years at the outpatient Hematology-Oncology Clinic of the Josephine Ford Cancer Institute, part of the Henry Ford Hospital and Health System. She is currently the Social Work Team Leader for the Josephine Ford Cancer Institute. She has been a Social Worker for a long time (don't even ask!!!), having previously worked at several other hospitals in the area. She also worked for 3 years as a Resident Service Coordinator in a HUD-subsidized senior congregate living apartment building, part of a larger group of congregate living buildings. She resides in Bloomfield Hills, MI. Her hobbies include reading, movies, and travel, when there is time, as well as spending time with her adult children (awaiting marriages and grandchildren someday!).

Susan M. Kocik, MSW, LICSW, retired as the social worker for people with bleeding disorders at the Hemophilia Care Program at the Puget Sound Blood Center in Seattle. She currently serves on the National Steering Committee of PEP (Parents Empowering Parents) and on the Board of Directors of the Bleeding Disorders Foundation of Washington. She lives in Seattle with her husband, Stephen Manes, and enjoys traveling, hiking, and reading.

Ed Kuebler, MSW, LCSW, has been employed at the Gulf States Hemophilia and Thrombophilia Treatment Center, Houston, TX, as the Social Services Coordinator for 15 years. He has worked in the bleeding disorders community for 20 years. He is a graduate of the University of Houston, Master of Social Work Graduate Program. Ed is currently the Director for the International PEP Training Program, Director for the Texas Summer Camp Leadership Program and Program Director for Step Up/ Reach Out (SURO) – An International Leadership Program. He developed and co-coordinates the Great Plains Regions' Annual Women with Bleeding & Clotting Disorders

Retreat. He is the co-author of a children's von Willebrands book called *Rafting Rescue: An Adventure at Camp Cascade.* He received the National Hemophilia Foundation's Social Worker of the Year Award in 2007. Ed is a member of the World Federation of Hemophilia Psychosocial Committee and a member of the National Hemophilia Foundation's "Steps for Living" task force.

Greg McClure, BA, MA, MS, LSW, is the father of two adult sons with hemophilia A. He has worked as an HTC social worker for over 12 years. He is retired from both the CNW/UP railroad (37 years) and the Michael Reese Hospital/RUSH Medical Center HTC's. Greg does volunteer work for the Hemophilia Federation of America, the National Hemophilia Foundation, COTT, the PEP program, and the Marcus McClure Big Dreams Foundation. He continues to educate and advocate for patients and their families with bleeding disorders.

Danna Merritt, MSW, LMSW, has been a social worker for over 40 years and the social worker for the Hemophilia Treatment Center located at Children's Hospital of Michigan in Detroit since 1987. Danna is the mother of two daughters, who, between them, have made her a proud grandmother five times since 2004. In addition to developing many other educational activities, programs, and psychosocial services these past 25 years, in 1996 she authored and now directs the well-known *Parents Empowering Parents* (PEP) program: a psychosocial intervention and parenting course for parents of children with bleeding disorders. During her years with the hemophilia community, she has felt privileged to witness the famous sociologist, Margaret Mead quote in action: "Never doubt that a small group of thoughtful, committed citizens can change the world; indeed, it's the only thing that ever has," as she has seen it in action in the hemophilia community. Empowering vs. enabling human beings is her passion, whether they are learning to ride a bike or facing the challenges inherent in living every aspect of their lives. Danna has learned much from those living with bleeding disorders during the past 25 years such as, but not limited to, valuable life lessons and the meaning of, and value in, strength of character when facing incredible challenges. Bottom line: with heartfelt thanks to all those patients and their families she's had the good fortune to work with in this community, she's learned how to take the "lemons" that come along in life and turn them into "lemonade!"

Hulda Niv, MSW, RSW, has 17 years of social work experience in the area of chronic illness including renal, diabetes, and bleeding disorders. During her employment at the Alberta Health Services, she has worked with multidisciplinary teams providing family-centered care services.

For the past seven years she has been working with the Hemophilia/Haematology/Immunology Clinic at the Alberta Children's Hospital. Her work with this population includes, but is not limited to, psychosocial assessments, providing education to patients and their families about inherited bleeding disorders, and counseling related to illness adjustment. Her focus with adolescents is on vocations, career choices, sexuality, transitioning, and self-esteem issues.

Laurel J. Pennick, MSSW, LCSW, is presently a clinical social worker at the Arizona Hemophilia and Thrombosis Center at the University of Arizona Health Sciences Center. Ms. Pennick has a 20 year plus history in the social work profession, including experience in Critical Care, Emergency and Trauma, ICU, Geriatric, Hospice, and seven years in Hemophilia Care. She has served as the social work representative for the National Hemophilia Foundation, chair of the NHF Social Work Working Group, and a member of MASAC. In her free time she is a tennis player, a hiker, a potter, a wife, and an adoptive mother of two very active adolescent cats.

Wayne Richards, MSW, LCSW, lives in Columbia, Missouri with his wife, Paula, a hospice social worker. He has almost 40 years of experience as a social worker, 10 of these as a medical social worker at the University of Missouri Hemophilia Treatment Center. Having retired, he now works part-time with the Walgreens Hemophilia Team. In the past, he served on the national Parents Empowering Parents Steering Committee and NHF's Social Work Working Group. He has two sons, both living in Kansas City, MO. One is a medical social worker and the other works for Brinks Armored Truck. His daughter and her husband are attorneys living in Phoenix, Arizona. He enjoys hiking, biking, and reading.

Bobbie Steinhart, MSW, was the social worker for the Hemophilia Treatment Center at Children's Hospital Oakland, for 20 years, until her retirement in 2003. She and her husband, Larry, live in Berkeley. Bobbie's a proud mother, mother-in-law and very involved grandmother of three young girls. In her free time, she's an avid walker, reader, quilter, enthusiastic cook, long-term volunteer in the Berkeley Public Schools, and, during election seasons, active in voter registration campaigns.

Silvia Vega, BA, has been a social services caseworker with the Hemostasis and Thrombosis Team at Children's Hospital Los Angeles (CHLA) for the past seven years. Prior to coming to the hemophilia community, she worked with Mental Health Services for five years and with the Dialysis and Renal Transplant teams. Her work has included both inpatient and outpatient care services. She has been working at CHLA since 1976. One of her interests has been facilitating support group meetings. As an adult student, she completed her B.A. degree in Interdisciplinary Studies from the University of Dominguez Hills in 2000. English is her second language. She is fluent in Spanish.

Dawn von Mayrhauser, MSW, LCSW, has been the social worker at the Connecticut Bleeding Disorders Center in Farmington, CT for 18 years. Before that, she worked in a home-based hospice program. She lives with her husband in West Hartford, CT, and has two grown sons. She loves reading fiction, mowing the lawn, and doing the Sunday New York Times crossword puzzle.